Tales from Mi

CW01431830

Claire Attwood

chipmunkapublishing
the mental health publisher

Claire Attwood

Published by
Chipmunkapublishing
PO Box 6872
Brentwood
Essex CM13 1ZT
United Kingdom

http://www.chipmunkapublishing.com

Chipmunkapublishing gratefully acknowledge the support of Arts Council England.

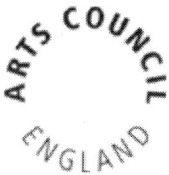

ARTS COUNCIL ENGLAND

Acknowledgements

I would like to thank all those people that have supported me and been there for me over the last 7 years, especially Neil, my parents Robin and Lynne, my sister Helen, brothers Mike and Steve, my grandmother Mary, and my mum-in-law Jackie and her husband Mike. Special thanks also to St Lucia, to my friend Lisa, and all my work colleagues who have encouraged me so much. Finally, I would like to thank Neil's nan-Vera, who is sadly no longer with us but was so supportive of my dream to have a book published.

Claire Attwood

Dedication

I would like to dedicate this book to my fiancé-Neil Smith.

Claire Attwood

DO I DARE?

This poem is about times when I felt that suicide was the only way out for me and the way that was 'offered' to me by the voices that I hear when I feel unwell. I often felt like this-I sometimes still do but the essence of this poem is about feeling cowardly for not going through with the act of suicide but then being able to take back control from the voices and realise my inner strength.

Whirling pools of darkness
Washing over me,
Take me far away from here,
Drown me in the sea.
Blood so red, it trickles
From my porcelain skin,
What is there to stop me now?
The ice is wearing thin.
And still I hear the voices,
Screaming through the air,
Do it, do it, do it
Am I brave enough to dare?

Standing on the precipice
Staring down to earth,
Want to end this all now
Break free from the curse.
Blood is flowing freely and
I start to slip away
What was once black and white
Fades to murky grey.
And still I hear the voices
Screaming through the air,
Do it, do it, do it,
Am I brave enough to dare?

Standing on the platform,
Waiting for a train,
Kill me, give me freedom,
Obliterate my brain.
Blood pours now so freely

From my heavy heart,
Life it ebbs away now
But is it just the start?
And still I hear the voices
Screaming through the air,
Do it, do it, do it!
Am I brave enough to dare?

Yet somehow through the darkness,
There comes a shining light,
Brings me back from the brink
Gives me second sight,
Blood no longer flows away,
I feel a strength within.
For this battle now is done,
Victorious! I win!
Where now are the voices
That once screamed through the air?
And now I know I'm brave enough
To live, to love, to care.

THE REAL ME?

This poem was written in frustration! I was doing quite well at dealing with my mental health problems but still felt incredibly vulnerable. Everyone around me seemed to have a lot of high expectations of me and I felt that I could never live up to these expectations. The road to recovery is seldom smooth...!

I really am not as thick-skinned
As people do assume.
Scaling the heights of ecstasy
Then trawling troughs of doom.
Yet people seem to expect me
To function just like them
I am scraping sub-zero
While they're a perfect ten!

And all the time they'll say to me,
Well done you've come so far
But in reality I feel
Like an alien from Mars!
They all think that I am strong
But how wrong could they be?
I feel my defences tumble down
I must not let them see!

And yes,I guess I mask it-
Probably very well
But for all this public heaven,
I live a private hell.
OK so things aren't quite as bad
As they used to be,
But people don't want to listen-
At least they don't to me.

I keep on ploughing forward
As there's no way back
But through my inner foundations
Appears a monstrous crack.
But no-one else can find it

I keep it hidden see
No-one ever wants to know
The loser that is me

Putting on the face again
My smile it feels so false
And no-one ever notices
I guess I'm just a fool.
I wish someone would listen
Just give me a chance
Please to help me move on
Don't want a song and dance!

I want to move on forward-
No point in looking back
See me for who I really am
And help me stay on track.
Remember- I have feelings,
Raw emotions too,
Support me when I need it
And never be untrue.

Remember I am damaged,
But I am human too.
The feelings that I have are real,
And influenced by you.
I really want to do the things
That other people can
But I need a little help-
Can you lend me a hand?

Tales from a Broken Mind

A MESSAGE FROM MR SARKY...

This poem was actually 'dictated' to me by a voice I hear (whom I call Mr Sarky).He told me this poem was a reflection of how my work colleagues saw me. Writing this left me feeling very emotionally drained but at the same time,it allowed me to externalise what the voice was saying.

I'm sorry you're not welcome,
So please now, go away!
I don't have time to speak to you
Not right now, not today!

You've got a lot to offer?
I don't believe a word.
You should just be silent-
Seen but never heard.

Please don't speak of heartbreak,
Don't really want to listen
And wipe those tears right off your face
I hate the way they glisten.

You say that you can do things
But really where's the proof?
You're getting on my nerves now-
Just go jump off the roof.

We'd be better off without you-
Things would run much smoother
If we didn't have to think about
You- psychotic loser.

Sit there in your corner,
Weep your silent tears,
Just don't bother me now,
Don't care about your fears.

No-one really wants you,
You're here just as a token.

You make the numbers balance right,
And leave the rules unbroken.

Don't ask us to have faith in you
Don't try to impress me.
Cos nothing that you say or do
Will change what I perceive.

Don't tell me of your background
No interest in your past.
We all wish that you'd just leave
And do it very fast.

We chose you,what a big mistake
And now we wish you'd go.
Just grab your things- return your keys,
Cos we don't want to know.

So stick your own experience
It really counts for nothing.
We all know far more than you,
Just go back to cutting.

Cos that's all that you are worth,
So watch your own blood flow
And let us all get on with it
We're the ones that know!

SECRET SHAME

This poem is about self-harm. I often felt relief from self-harming as it seemed to appease Mr Sarky -but- it was only very short-lived relief because after that comes the guilt and the intense feeling of shame. I felt this shame at two levels. Firstly I felt shame for damaging something as unbroken and precious as my own skin all at the command of a voice and secondly because society takes a dim view of those of us who have self-injured. My hope is that people who know someone who self-harms,will read this and begin to understand just how it feels to do this to oneself. Maybe then,people who self-harm will be understood and treated with kindness rather than the disgrace and humiliation that they often face.

You see my bloodied wound
And sense physical pain
But the guilt that burns beneath
Fuels my secret shame.

You think I can just stop
And place on me the blame
If only 'twas so simple
To kill my secret shame.

Living on the razor's edge,
A face without a name
Soon there'll be another scar
For my secret shame.

My skin is torn and ragged
My sleeve is red again
But now relief is all I feel
Until my secret shame.

To you it's such a stupid act
Attention seeking game
But you will never understand
About my secret shame.

A great big disappointment

Claire Attwood

It goes against the grain
To harm such perfect skin this way
It's called my secret shame.

Another ruined chance to prove
That we are all the same
I deal with things in my own way
And it's my secret shame.

I know that it's dysfunctional
Wild and never tame
But must you always turn your backs
On my secret shame?

I want to stop I really do
And break free from these chains
So try to empathise with me
And heal my secret shame.

DEMONS

This poem was written in a great deal of anger after I was sent to see a woman from a free-church as it was believed that I was demon-possessed. I was not demon-possessed at all but living with psychosis that I was keeping to myself as I was too frightened to seek help.

They told me I had demons
Devils in my head
That just had to be exorcised
Or I would end up dead.

They sent me to a lady
A person I once knew
To get rid of the 'demons'
And my mind to screw.

She sat me in an armchair
In the middle of the room
And spoke to me of hell-fire
And prophecies of doom.

She hovered hands above my head
And claimed to speak in tongues
But she made me scream out loud,
From the bottom of my lungs!

Freaky,scary,weird and odd
Emotions that I had
I never had a demon
I was just going mad!

I am not demon possessed
And nor was I ever
So trying to exorcise something
'twas not very clever!

ALL I EVER WANTED...

This poem is about my experiences of being bullied at school because I was a little 'different'. I now know that the reason I was 'different' was because of my developing psychosis.

Oh to be part of the gang
The popular kids at school
Always on the outside
Excluded like a fool.

And all I ever wanted was acceptance-was that too much to ask?

Standing on the outside
Trying to look in
Sick of playing loser
I just want to win

And all I ever wanted was acceptance-was that too much to ask?

Success shone all around me
Wanted to claim my part
But fate snatched it away-
A knife-blow to the heart.

And all I ever wanted was acceptance-was that too much to ask?

So if you see a sad kid
At the circle's edge
Invite her to join in somehow
She'd be grateful if you did.

Cos all she ever wanted was acceptance-was that too much to ask?

CRYIN' AGAIN

This poem was written about the long, lonely and unhappy nights that I used to spend crying. I found that my problems always felt worse at night and because I was trying to fight the psychosis alone, night time when everyone else was asleep, was the only time I felt I could express my deep unhappiness. Though this only served to make me feel more alone and isolated than ever before.

Sat alone at night again
The whole world is asleep
On the bathroom floor I sit
And I begin to weep.

The tears pouring down again
From my bloodshot eyes
I try to stay silent
So no-one hears my cries.

Drowning in my tears again
Wishin' I was dead
Free me from my pain
Release me from my head.

Sinking under pain again
No-one seems to care
This destroys my soul
But help it is nowhere.

Shut up!They shout again
I'm keeping them awake
No attempts to comfort me
Just shut up for F#*k's sake!

Feeling bitterness again
No-one wants to know
Want to get away from life
But got no place to go.

So I'll cry in the bathroom again

And try to hide my fears
Don't want to disturb them
With my futile tears.

And I 'll learn to cope again
With the prison that's my brain
Try to stop cryin' again
Silently go insane.

LOOK AT HER!

This poem is about the running commentary that I sometimes experience from Mr Sarky (a voice I hear).It becomes very annoying and it usually leaves me in a very bad mood when this happens.

Look at her! That girl there
Walking down the street
Bet she'll fall or stumble
Trip over her own feet!

Look at her! That girl there
Tryin' to appear
As normal as the rest of us?
Nah!She's freakin' weird!

Look at her! That girl there
Actin' like she's cool
Concealing her madness
She just looks a fool!

Look at her! That girl there
Talkin' to herself
Keepin' high and dry now
Or left upon the shelf?

Look at her! That girl there
We have complete control
Over everything she does
Her life's like a black hole.

Look at her! That girl there
We kick her when she's down
Remind yourself to spit on her
If you see her around town!

Look at her! That girl there
Don't give her time of day
Be as cruel as you like

And perhaps she'll fade away......

WATCHING ME

This poem is about the feeling that I sometimes have when I am feeling unwell. I feel like I have some kind of microchip inside my brain, put there by the Government so that they can spy on me. I know that may sound ridiculous, but when I am feeling unwell, it becomes very real- and very frightening.

You can never see them
But believe me they are there
Watching every move I make
I wish I didn't care.

I sense them all around me
Messin' with my head
And if they ever catch me
I know I'll end up dead.

All around me they are there
Governmental spies
Just cos I can't see them
Doesn't mean they've got no eyes.

Conversing with my spy chip
Taking over me
Reporting back to HQ
Everything they see.

Thinkin' they could lull me
Instil in me some trust
But that will never happen
they turned my brain to mush.

Wishin' they couldn't see
All that's in my head
One day I'll rebel 'gainst them
And I'll shoot them dead!

But until then I must survive
Knowing that they're there

Hide myself away from them
Deny them of a share!

WHAT YOU DON'T SEE...

This poem is again one written out of frustration at people thinking
everything is ok with me when inside, I am struggling.

You think it's almost over
But it's only just begun
All that's left is darkness
No hope of the sun.

Look at me-what is there?
Behind the cool facade
Happiness does not exist
It's all a big charade.

You say you can't believe it
That I look so damn good
But my emotions now are numb
Just like old, dead wood.

You reckon I'm successful,
I turned my life around.
But all my hope has vanished
Buried underground.

You can't see my anguish
I disguise all my pain
But when I sit here all alone,
It pours like acid rain.

You all think I'm happy
You cannot see my fears
You only hear my laughter
You do not see my tears.

So please try to remember
When you see me grin
My face it hides the pain I feel
The pain that is within.

ILLUSIONS/DELUSIONS?

This poem is written about hallucinations or,as I prefer to call them, extra-special life perceptions (ESPLs for short).When I see or hear things that others around me do not, it is very easy for others to say "it's just an hallucination" but is it? Who is to say what exists and what doesn't?

I see the world around me
Differently from you
But just cos I see things that you can't
Doesn't mean that they're untrue.

I see people in the walls
Whom you never perceive
But I know that they exist
Why can't you just believe?

It really is amazing!
That's why I stop and stare-
At things that you just cannot see
Like faces in thin air.

You tell me that it's all not real
And say that I am ill
If only you could see them
It's really quite a thrill!

You all think I am crazy
You say I'm going mad
But I don't really think I am
Your words make me feel sad.

I can sometimes see things
Like patterns in the sky
A patchwork quilt of beauty
Draped on clouds so high

I often hear pure music
A secret symphony
You all nod or shake your heads

Tales from a Broken Mind

In shrouded sympathy.

I hear fabulous ideas
That echo through my head
But it's all a secret-
All the things they said

And you will never believe me
You say it's a delusion
But I know it's me that's real
And you that's an illusion.

UNLUCKY YOU

This poem was written about my experiences at school. None of the other kids wanted to sit next to me because they all thought I was freaky and weird. They used to say how unlucky they felt if the teacher told them that they had to sit next to me. What they didn't realise was that I felt just as unlucky as they did because I had to sit next to them!

Unlucky you they said
You have to sit by Freak-Girl
Cos teacher told you that you must
And now you just want to hurl!

Unlucky you they said
Stuck there with her freakiness
No choice in the matter
Infected by her geekiness

Unlucky you they said
Sharing desk space with the Freak
Her weirdness it is catching
You'll be mad within a week!

Unlucky you they said
You can't escape ol' Freaky
She sits there crying all day long
Her face all pale and streaky.

Unlucky you they said
What about poor ol' Freak-Girl?
She's unfortunate you see
Stuck in her painful world.

Unlucky you they said
Please be kind to Freak-Girl
For she's the lonely one you see
In a sad unhappy world.

UNWANTED ATTENTION

This poem was written about someone who gave me unwanted attention and completely overstepped boundaries that should never be crossed. I think that it is self-explanatory.

A venomous kiss
The kiss of death
I can almost smell it now
Putrid on his breath

A hand reaching too far
Fear inside my heart
Just leave me alone now
In his web I'm caught

Take away my liberty
Feeling panic rise
Get your hands right off me
Anger in his eyes

I sit here alone again
Yet somehow I feel dirty
Was it all my fault tonight?
Did I act all flirty?

Did I bring this on myself?
Did I give him the come on?
Feeling like I want to die
All my strength,I summon.

I feel so bloody angry
But I feel frightened too
His roaming hands they scare me
And revolt me too.

So take your dirty hands off
I am not yours to touch
You'll never hurt me again
At least not quite as much.

THE EVER-PRESENT MR SARKY

This poem was written about Mr Sarky and how he is always with me-usually annoying or upsetting me.

You look at me through dusk, through dawn
It's clear that you despise me.
You look at me- it's daggers drawn
At least that's what my eyes see!

You comfort me with hollow lies
I know that you are scheming.
I've seen it all with my own eyes
Don't tell me I am dreaming!

You think that I don't understand
That I can't see right through you
You're conniving and you're underhand
Evil through and through!

You hound me and you haunt me so
I don't know where to turn
You kick me when I'm feeling low
And mock me as I burn.

You're in my ear the whole damned day
You never let me rest
Until the time I fade away
You won't give up your quest.

You will never let me go
'Til my hopes have all but faded
Burned in the fire's icy glow
Broken, burnt and jaded.

You make me feel so bad inside
And steal all my self-worth
You've hated me- laughed as I cried
From the moment of my birth.

So go on then despise me

cos I no longer care
I've lived with you beside me
My life a grim nightmare.

But I'll keep on fighting
And I'll win this war
You can keep on biting
I am scared of you no more.

SOLITUDE

This poem was written about feeling lonely and isolated-cut off from the world. But while I was secretly battling my psychosis,solitude was an escape for me to get away from the rest of the world that I found unbearably threatening.

Solitude oh solitude
My dearest lonely friend!
Solitude oh solitude
On you I can depend.

Solitude oh solitude
Descend on me like rain
Solitude oh solitude
Echoes of my pain.

Solitude oh solitude
Break my fragile skin
Solitude oh solitude
Free the beast within.

Solitude oh solitude
Bitter sweet thou art!
Solitude oh solitude
Mend my broken heart.

Solitude oh solitude
Over me you cascade
Solitude oh solitude
With you,all night,I prayed.

Solitude oh solitude
Free me from your spell
Solitude oh solitude
Release me from my cell.

THIEF

This particular poem was written retrospectively,about the years that
my psychosis 'stole' from me.

Watch my heart beat out of time
Battered, bruised, broken, burned
And tell me what you got from it
The hardest truth you ever learned.

Watch my eyes flicker with pain
Harmed, hurt, harrowed, hard
And show me what you stole from them
I was fragile,dropped my guard.

See my lips they quiver so
Terrorised, torn, tortured, taut
And whisper what you took from them
The stolen silence that you sought.

See my skin so spoiled now
Ruined, rotten, raw, ravaged
And give me what you gained from it
The life you thieved and savaged.

And tell me when you see me cry
You feel a pang of guilt
For like a flower you cut me down
And left me there to wilt.

Claire Attwood

THIS SPECIAL GIFT OF MINE

This poem is a bit of fun really as it discusses the positive aspects of experiences commonly called hallucinations.

I see faces in thin air
And patterns on the wall
You must be mad they all declare
Or else some kind of fool!

I see people atop the clouds
And designs in the sky
They bury themselves in sanity's shrouds
I've often wondered why!

For is it not a gift of mine
Akin to luck or magic
'Tis they who lack something divine
And that, I feel, is tragic!

So next time that you see me,
Staring into space
Don't label me as crazy
For my gift I'll not waste.

DON'T WANT TO KNOW...

This poem is about feeling deeply unhappy and unsupported.

I have a sneaking feeling
I really need to cry
I know it's not appealing
But please don't ask me why.

I know that I should try to
Learn to push it under
But every time I see you
I cannot help but wonder.

You say it's 'just' emotion
And I should deal with it
Give me a magic potion
So I don't feel a bit!

You don't want to see me cry
But not because you care
You can't bear to see damp cheeks
Of tears you want no share.

I refuse to push it under
Bottle it up today
Because,in case you wonder
I do not need your say!

And if you're feeling sad now
I'm afraid it's just hard luck
For being so uncaring-
You couldn't give a ....

SHIPMATES

This is a poem I wrote when I was feeling quite good in terms of my mood-hence the humorous element of it.

The sea crashes onto the shore
The tide it is a-turning
But I am trapped behind the door
My every fibre yearning.

The Cap'n hollers "Land ahoy!"
The voyage almost through now
But it was just a subtle ploy
An iceberg tears the bow!

The ship it is a-sinkin'
Not quite sure what to say
Should I waste time thinkin'?
Or try to swim away?

I suppose we've all been lucky
We had our pleasure cruise
But I don't feel so plucky
When my life I could lose!

But they all laugh aloud at me
As I sink beneath the water
Neptune's revenge- the dark cold sea
Like I'm Medusa's daughter!

I feel myself begin to drown
I'm being pulled right under
And in my head the biggest sound
Of angry Mars' thunder!

Body and soul now separates
I hope I'll get to Heaven
No thanks to my old ship-mates
No lucky number seven!

And if I am in purgatory

Tales from a Broken Mind

For a substantial time
Restore me to my former glory
I committed no crime!

Remember all the so-called friends
Who were just hangers-on?
On them you just cannot depend
Forget me now I'm gone...

LITTLE BIRD

This poem is written about my Grandmother who has Dementia. It describes her frailty and how it feels as though she has been taken from us even though she is still here with us.

I hold you in my hand
Little broken bird
Scooped up from cold cruel sand
A whisper of a word.

Your feathers are all spattered
With heavy acrid oil
Yet no-one thought it mattered
Your body ripped and soiled.

For life was mean and hard on you
And crushed your tiny beak
Took your life, obscured your view
Stole your right to speak.

Light extinguished from your eyes
No longer shall they glisten
Thieves, they spun a web of lies
And forced your ears to listen.

Your broken wings no longer flutter
But they twitch so feebly
'Twas once a song but now a mutter
They acquired deceitfully.

Dearest little broken bird
I leave you now to rest
Remembering the songs I heard
When you were at your best.

LAKESIDE LAMENT

This poem is about feeling excluded by people and being unable to
appreciate the beauty around me as everything seemed so bleak
when I was in deep depression.

The lake it rippled beneath the moonlight
And willow trees softly sighed
While I stood there just out of sight
All alone with the tears I cried.

The sheer beauty of the water lily
And the graceful gliding swans
Yet I stood there feeling silly
For everyone else had gone.

And I waded through the icy water,
My feet tangled in the reeds
Like a lamb awaiting slaughter
Whose cries nobody heeds.

As I crept among the silver fishes
Past a solitary duck,
I won't waste my time on wishes
As I never had much luck.

I trample softly underneath my feet
The lazy picnic's litter
My heart finding it hard to beat
My soul is oh so bitter.

I find no solace in this beauty
The treasure I seek, forlorn
I have more than paid my dues
From the moment I was born.

DARKNESS

This poem was written with reference to the way I used to stay
awake most of the night as everyone else had gone to bed and I
could sneak downstairs and cry without disturbing anyone.

Darkness cold, cold darkness
Oh come envelope me
Take me from this world so cruel
For you can set me free.

Darkness cold, cold darkness
I beg you- hear my cry
Break the chains that bind me so
And let me up to fly.

Darkness cold, cold darkness
Come on devour me
Let me savour my release
Whilst no-one else can see.

Darkness cold, cold darkness
Conceal me in your shroud
While all is dead around me
This silence feels too loud.

Darkness cold, cold darkness
My comforting palindrome
Take me far away from here
To my spiritual home.

NO 'I' IN TEAM?

This poem was written about a place where I used to work.
Whenever I tried to express any personal feelings about the job we
were doing, another person used to quip-"there's no I in team".
I quickly came back with an answer-that although the letter I is not
found in team, the letters M and E are! I have always maintained
that in order for any team to function well, the components have to
be happy. This poem is a bit of fun based on that idea!

There is no 'I' in team you say
And I guess that much is true
But if you look you'll find M E
And that's important too!

For if a team is to work well
The components must be good
To run things as clear as a bell
To do what a team should.

So if you're sitting there thinking
All about what you should do
How to stop a team from sinking
Remember me and not just you!

For if a team is to work out
In a reasonable fashion
There is no room for your doubt
No matter how strong the passion!

So before you turn around to see
And remind me there's no I
Remember that there is a me...
In team without an 'I'!

A LEAP OF FAITH

This one is all about recovery and how it is like a journey. There
have been times in my life when my recovery journey has been
interrupted but that's just how it goes. Recovery can be a scary thing
as you have to confront and challenge the ways in which you
approach life and the way in which you think. In short, recovery is
hard work but I think it's worth it!

I took the quantum leap of faith
Not knowing what I'd find
A stab in the dark, a gamble
Be still my frightened mind!

A dive into the deep unknown
There was no guarantee
The only one to rely on
I found out, fast, was me!

It felt like I was blindfolded
And left there in the dark
So I learned to fight it alone
The outlook though, was stark.

But still I carried on fighting
Cos life is sink or swim
I chose swim, as to choose sink
Would be extremely dim!

I refuse to play the victim
For what's the point in that?
It renders you so dis-empowered
The subject of idle chat!

I will keep on climbing upwards
Never will I stop
The only way is up you see
Until you reach the top.

If on my way, I trip or fall
Or take a little tumble

Tales from a Broken Mind

I'll dust myself off and try again
For it was only a stumble.

And I will fear not the pot-holes
The road's many twists and turns
For that's how I'll recover
And live and grow and learn.

And I'll keep on walking onward
In deepest night or day
For life is never black or white
But various shades of grey.

INSANE,INSANE,INSANE!

This poem was written about (some of) the names people call those of us with mental health problems. It is quite humorous as I think bigots find it hard to be laughed at by the objects of their derision!

You might think I'm crazy
But that's alright with me
What you see is what you get
Fools' words come easily.

You might think I'm bonkers
As mad as mad could be
But it doesn't bother me now
For I have been set free!

You might think I'm nutty
A fruitcake-that's okay
For when you close that mouth of yours
Your words just fade away!

You might think I'm crackers
Touched by insanity
But go look in the mirror
Cos it might not just be me!

You might think I'm mental
But you are just a pain
For who are you to label me?
Insane, insane, insane!

MR SARKY'S TAKEOVER

This poem is written about Mr Sarky and the way in which he sneaks up on me and tries to take over.

Poison courses through my veins
As Mr Sarky takes the reins
It's like a bullet to the brain
And only I can feel the pain

Resistance spells futility
Through my own stupidity
Try to win back my liberty
Before I reach senility

Now the venom starts to seize
Grips me like a vile disease
Makes me fall to my knees
Release me Mr Sarky please.

I violently start to shake
Is it really real or fake?
Am I sleeping or awake?
Mr Sarky for F's sake!

Grinding my face in the dirt
Knowing it will really hurt
Tearing my best T-shirt
His fury to assert.

I know I cannot win
So do I just give in?
That would be a sin
Not doing anythin'

So I guess I'll fight
And use all my might
I will be all right
Second time tonight!

Mr Sarky you just leave!
No more me to deceive
I will never believe
My life I shall retrieve!

And now he's gone
Stopped goin' on
The sun it shone
La vie-c'est bon!

WHEN I'M GONE

This poem is all about feeling suicidal and also angry that the actions and inactions of others made me feel that way. It also explores how death can seem very inviting when life is too hard to bear.

I'm sick of this exclusion
Of feeling ripped and torn
This icy cold seclusion
My own passing I now mourn.
Nothing but isolation
And feeling all alone
No cause for celebration
My soul has been disowned.

Little dark spirit
Flying round the room
Hovers on my shoulder
I sense impending doom.

All around me is confusion
About who I really am
Or am I just an illusion
As people pass me by?
A truly heartfelt scream now
Tears open my throat
I scream for you to save me
But there is no antidote.

Little dark spirit
Flying round the room
Hovers on my shoulder
I sense impending doom.

And will this ever leave me?
Or am I marked for life?
A world where people don't see
Beyond war and strife
No one seems to give a damn

About the chaos building
And no one cares who I am
When power they are wielding.

Little dark spirit
Flying round the room
Hovers on my shoulder
I sense impending doom.

As terror grips my voice now
Impossible to speak
I've done the encore and the bow
The coffin lid,it creaks
And all because nobody cared
Enough to give me room
I'm lying here so cold and scared
Interred within my tomb.

Little dark spirit
Flying round the room
Hovers on my shoulder
I sense impending doom.

The grave looks so inviting
As I sink beneath the soil
Death is not exciting
But nor is life's hard toil
The ones who used to give me grief
Now?I just ignore 'em.
Goodbyes from them were oh so brief
No dents in their decorum!

Little dark spirit
Flying round the room
Hovers on my shoulder
I sense impending doom.

And as they turn and walk away
From my final resting place
They live to see another day
I sample God's good grace

Tales from a Broken Mind

So if you see them joking
Remind them please of I
Their consciences need poking
They'll know precisely why.

LITTLE BLUE PILL

This poem was written in a fit of anger. I was angry at having to rely on medication to keep me on an even keel. It also has elements of denial-or is it enlightenment(?) in it as I sometimes have phases where I don't believe it's an illness at all but is just another way of viewing the world and that I experience the world on a different level sometimes. It feels like a blessing and a curse all rolled into one.

Little blue pill
You make me ill
When I'm as right as rain
Little blue pill
I am not ill
Cure non-existent pain

Little blue pill
You make me ill
Forcing me to swallow
Little blue pill
I am not ill
Your victory is hollow.

Little blue pill
You make me ill
Giving me no choice
Little blue pill
I am not ill
Yet no one heard my voice.

Little blue pill
You make me ill
And try to make me sleep
Little blue pill
I am not ill
Yet you make me weep.

Little blue pill
You make me ill
When there is nothing wrong

Tales from a Broken Mind

Little blue pill
I am not ill
And still you did me wrong.

Little blue pill
You make me ill
But you've had your day
Little blue pill
I am not ill
As I flush you away..

Claire Attwood

A HAPPY ENDING...

This poem was written following the funeral of my Fiance Neil's
Nan. I guess it helped me cope with the grief of losing her as I was
very close to her and loved her very much.

Weep not for me when I am gone
 I'll not be far away
For where the golden sun has shone
Cometh another day

Stand not in sadness at my grave
for I reside not there
and when our friendship you do crave
whisper me a prayer

Wring not your hands nor bow your head
As my cortege passes by
remember me alive-not dead
Please promise me you'll try.

Sink not into death's deep despair
in darkness seek only light
For I have pain no more to bear
God's love restores my sight.

Cry not nor abandon hope
For our love will endure
And God will teach you how to cope
Of this you can be sure.

So please be strong,shed not a tear
For I'm in paradise
I'll see you there so have no fear
I live eternal life.

THIS CRAZY LIFE

This is a crazy little poem that I wrote when I was feeling more than
somewhat hyper!

This crazy life it drives me mad
I'm going up the wall
Like Humpty Dumpty and his men
About to have a fall!

This crazy life it drives me mad
it makes me feel quite ill
When Jack fell down he broke his crown
But what became of Jill?

This crazy life it makes me mad
I feel just like a puppet
No spider though,scares me away
Apologies to Miss Muffet!

This crazy life it makes me mad
I don't know where I am
When sound asleep I lost my sheep
And Mary's little lamb!

This crazy life it drives me mad
I don't know what to do
I've fallen out with Bo Peep
And the old woman and her shoe.

This crazy life it drives me mad
Things they go too far
So I'll go and stare at the sky
Twinkle little star.

TO NEIL

This is a poem for my Fiance Neil whom I love so much.

How did we fall in love so deep
It almost feels divine
I guess we'll never really know
Our paths seemed to entwine

I lovingly gaze into your eyes
Devotion's what I find
You've stuck by me through thick and thin
Even when I lost my mind.

My love for you it is so strong
We'll never be apart
For I love you more and more
With each beat of my heart.

I look at you and feel a tingle
Running through my spine
The best thing is that I am yours
And you are also mine.

As wrinkles creep upon our faces
And we grow old and grey
Tomorrows are in short supply
But we'll always have today.

HE IS NOT A PART OF ME

Again, this is an angry poem written after yet another person told me that a voice I hear, was an extension of myself. I was very upset and angry as I would never say 90% of what this voice says to me to anyone- including myself. I do find it immensely frustrating when people who have never heard voices, try to tell those of us that have heard them what they are and where they come from.

A silent tear prickles,
And threatens to drown me
Running down my face,
Fleeing angry eyes.
It started in my mind
Then he got hold of it
My thoughts were not my own.
He put them there.

Nobody believes me,
But I know the truth.
He is not a part of me
Why can't people see that?
He is a separate entity.
He and I are not the same being,
Yet still people continue
Putting the blame on me,
Saying he's my unconscious incarnate
But they don't know the truth.
They make assumptions
About my sanity-say I'm crazy,
Only I know the truth.
And he is NOT a part of me.

Claire Attwood

LITTLE FICKLE TRICKLE

Another poem about how the voices taunt and torment me.

Little fickle trickle
How you infiltrate my brain
Making me feel crazy
Driving me insane.

Little fickle trickle
You're overwhelming me
Stealing both of my eyes
Ruling what I see.

Little fickle trickle
Now you're doing it again
Making me unhappy
Drowning me in pain.

Little fickle trickle
What makes you act so cruel?
You see that I am hurting
Yet treat me as a fool!

Little fickle trickle
To you it may be such fun
To kiss and then to slap me
Then shoot me with your gun!

Little fickle trickle
Why won't you set me free?
Poison me from the inside.
Hang me from a tree.

Little fickle trickle
Your words-they are just lies
To make me feel unwell
Slashing me like knives.

Little fickle trickle
What the hell is going on?

Tales from a Broken Mind

You're killing me-I can't breathe
Too late now, I am gone......

NEGATIVE SPIRAL

This one is all about the mood component of Schizoaffective disorder. It explains how I start at the top of the spiral and things go rapidly downhill from there onwards until I reach the bottom. The good thing is that once you've reached rock bottom, the only way is upwards!

You start at the top
That's where it begins
But this is a game
Where nobody wins

The spiral of life
Takes a downward turn
You fall ever faster
Then crash and burn.

I call it the spiral
For that's what it is
Go spinning down further
Cos life is a swizz.

Nobody to help you
No-one to care
The old adage proffered
'Life isn't fair'.

And still you keep falling
You're tumbling down
But nobody hears you
Your scream has no sound.

As depression grips you
In it's icy hand
Is this what it's come to?
It's not what I planned.

The feelings take over
You lose all control
Spiralling down now

Tales from a Broken Mind

Into the black hole.

You're caught in a current
A huge tidal wave
It crushes the hopes
That you always crave.

The light is extinguished
The flame it expires
No hopes for the future
No spark in your eyes.

Where has the hope gone
Where is the passion
You've fallen from grace
In spectacular fashion.

Yet somewhere inside you
There lies hidden power
You have such strength
No flames can devour.

And slowly you pick up
and upwards you grow
Cos when you've hit rock bottom
You can't go more low.

So climb the hill steadily
Ascend like no other
And with genuine hope
I know you'll recover.

So next time you find yourself
at the start of that spiral
Just try and think positive
To ensure your survival.

LIFE'S JOURNEY

This is about how life is like a journey with all it's little twists and turns etc.

Life is a journey
A road which we travel
And in it are problems
Our lives to unravel

Sometimes it is uphill
Sometimes it is down
But we keep on walking
Till happiness is found.

We encounter pot holes
We stumble on bumps
But still we move onwards
Till we come up trumps.

And when bad things happen
Or things don't go our way
We still keep on going
For guidance we pray.

And as we walk on forwards
As we keep going forth,
We follow the track before us
Be it east,south,west or north.

Sometimes we stagger up the hill
And other times we stride
But we'll keep going onwards
For we've nothing to hide.

DISILLUSIONMENT

This poem was written when I was feeling very depressed with life.

When you cannot see any clear conclusion
Is it any wonder you feel disillusioned?

When the sun won't rise and the moon won't fall
Craving a breeze but there's nothing at all.

When you feel this sickening yearning
The ice melted and the fire's now burning.

When deep inside your own dead mind
No sweet, sweet solace can you ever find.

When your reputation's been dragged through mud
It pollutes your soul and poisons your blood.

When you stumble where you used to swagger
Knife in the back, a bitter, cold dagger.

When you are rejected by the whole wide world
Is it any wonder that you come unfurled?

When being yourself is all that matters
Who cares if the whole world shatters.........

EXCLUDE ME

This poem is about the exclusion those of us with mental health problems often encounter. Basically it is a reflection of the ignorance of some people.

The papers shout it- "New" "Exclusive"!!
But I am just an old reclusive.
I will hide away in my home
Crawl under the nearest stone.

For I am now called deluded
No use, crap, dumped, excluded.
So I will try hard to disappear
I'll not be back so have no fear.

Label me, another weird psychosis
No more hope-a dark prognosis.
Another one mad, schizo, weird
Treat me like I should be feared.

Turn it round-you're affected
Cut me out, make me feel rejected.
Poke fun at me, go on and laugh
Another schizo, she must be daft.

Tell the world-lets start a rumour
And watch it grow like a tumour.
Look at me-what a bloody state
I see your eyes glazed with hate.

I didn't turn out quite as expected
So that's why I am disrespected.
And in all of this confusion
All I get is damned exclusion.

EXTRA SPECIAL LIFE PERCEPTION

Sometimes, I think that people who don't see visions or hear voices,
are actually missing out on an exciting dimension of life. I know
that a lot of the time I experience negative voices and visions, but
sometimes I feel that the good stuff makes up for those bad ones!

Wow there! Did you just see that?
A multi coloured psychedelic cat!
Did you see her fibre-optic whiskers?
Man! I can't believe you missed her!

Amazing! Look did you catch it?
An entire city inside my crisp packet!
Streets, houses, people, cars
You look at me as if I were from Mars!

Hey there! Did you just watch it?
I saw this lamp post launch a rocket!
Maybe it's on it's way to go fishing
You guys don't know what you're missing!

Crikey! What d'you mean you missed it?
 I saw a frog prince and I kissed it!
Now I'll live in a prince's palace
Yet you won't drink from my chalice.

Blimey! How is it you can't see?
The same amazing world as me?
You say that I am hallucinating,
I should not keep ruminating.

But you will never understand,
I see a very different land.
You all think that I am mad.
But your lack of insight is oh so sad.

The world that only I see
Is filled with infinite beauty.
It's a shame that you just cannot see

The things that mean so much to me.

THE CHIP

This is another one about the chip I sometimes believe is inside my brain.

I have this chip inside my brain
That's the reason I'm insane
Or so I'm told by those that know
The news came as a bitter blow.

The government they put it there
It's true they did-I'm sure-I swear.
And so my mind can be quite hazy
As I sit here going crazy.

Implanted when I was a child
And still they ask why I was wild!
A 'watched' one, indeed I surely am
They watch me via their brain-cam!

They try to program my ideas
Expose me to my deepest fears
Control me to the nth degree
From them will I ever be free?

They steal my thoughts and read my mind
Leaving me helpless, lonely and blind.
They work on me dark wizardry
And leave me in abject misery.

One injustice to another
Don't blame my father or my mother
For they truly did never know
How those in power could stoop so low.

So I apologise if one day I flip
And tear out my brain-and the chip
At least in death I will be free
For they'll no longer spy on me!

MR SARKY

This is a bit of an angry outburst, directed at Mr Sarky for upsetting me...again.

Feckless fool!
Heartless, cruel!
Yet no-one ever sees you!

Nasty, mean!
Never seen!
And only I perceive you!

Evil, bad!
Crazy, mad!
I always feel your presence!

Wicked, lies!
Hate, despise!
You are never pleasant!

Vile, you liar!
Insipid fire!
I wish I never knew you!

Repulsed, hurt!
Rotten, dirt!
I'd run a blade right through you!

Beaten, bruised!
Cold, abused!
You think you are so glorious!

Alive, new?
Free of you?
One day I'll be victorious!

LIFE STORM

This poem compares my experiences of life to the weather.

A crashing crack of thunder
The rain begins to pour
I scream as I go under
Just can't take any more.

A stormy strike of lightning
Flashes across the sky
The world, it feels so frightening
And nobody knows why.

A rampant, raging rush of wind
Rips right through my skin
Punish me for I have sinned
The excuse is wearing thin.

A horrid, howling hurricane
Tears right through my mind
I want freedom from this pain
But life is seldom kind.

The torrid, teeming rain storm
It ravages my heart
I long for once to feel warm
I crave a fresh new start.

TEARS

Fairly self-explanatory, this one is all about crying.

If tears were like rivers
That flow to the sea,
I'd unleash the shivers
That overwhelm me.

If tears were like oceans
That move with the swell
I'd live with the notion
This sadness to quell.

If tears were like raindrops
That fall from the sky
I'd let all the pain stop
And in relief, sigh.

If tears were like great lakes
That reflect beauty
I'd struggle for their sakes
And do my duty.

If tears were like puddles
There at the roadside
I'd still cause these muddles
My guilt not denied.

If tears were like dark seas
That threaten my life
I'd surrender to siege
Yet still hold the knife.

If tears were like cool streams
I'd sit by their side
And indulge in my dreams
Till the time they all lied.

If tears were like torrents
That fall from the sky

I'd ask if it warrants
Another one to die.

SPIES

This is all about feeling watched- but with a dash of humour!

They spy on me,
I know they do-
What you don't know
Is they watch you too!

A camera here
Surveillance there
Those private moments
You don't want to share!

The walls have ears
The cameras eyes
But you can't see them
For they are disguised!

Government watchers
All of them liars
Light another match
On the funeral pyres.

For the world is a stage
And we are but players
But this world operates
On different layers.

So please be so cautious
In whatever you do
Cos right now those spies
Are preying on you!

DISEMPOWERMENT

This one was written in anger at people paying lip-service to including me in things but not really being interested in what I had to say.

You invite me to speak
Yet heed not my voice
You instruct me to choose
Yet give me no choice

You enquire how I feel
Yet don't empathise
You question what I see
Yet obscure my eyes

You ask my opinion
Yet still shout me down
You glare when I'm laughing
Yet smile when I frown

You query what I'm thinking
Yet pay no attention
You take all the praise
Yet give me no mention

You promise me some respect
Yet treat me like dirt
You ask why I'm crying
Yet dismiss my hurt

You tell me you'll listen
Yet I repeat words again
You offer no comfort
Yet you see I'm in pain

You should inspire hope
Yet you cause me to despair
You've time for the world
Yet no time for Claire.

SENSATION

Another poem about Mr Sarky and how much of an effect he has on my life.

I feel his acrid, rancid breath
On the back of my vulnerable neck
The smell of doom, despair and death
My life, he endeavours to wreck.

I sense his icy fingers point
At past things best forgotten
My sanity, he will disjoint
Leaving me so wretched and rotten.

I see his demons on the walls
Within which I am imprisoned
My life, it has been plagued with fools
Not the wonder I'd envisaged.

I hear his hurtful, hateful tones
That echo right through my brain
He leaves me crying all alone
Taunts me until I go insane.

I smell his frightful, putrid stench
He threatens to devour me
As I lay buried in a trench
He has disempowered me

I taste the bitterness of death
That all pervading flavour
And as I draw my final breath
I cry out for my saviour.

But when I'm gone-it's too late
To apologise for all the wrongs
Cos I'll be there at Heaven's gate
You'll see I was right all along!

NEGATIVE-POSITIVE

This one is all about how people can really affect the mood of others just by being either positive or negative.

Tease me, taunt me
Do your worst
Hurt me, haunt me
I am cursed.

Punch me, slap me
Break my heart
Grab me, trap me
Torn apart.

Hate me, harm me
Go ahead
Fool me, charm me
I am dead.

Find me, catch me
Whatever
Bite me, scratch me
Forever.

Throw me, lose me
On the heap
Wound me, bruise me
Sadness creeps.

Or............

Help me, heal me
Be my friend
Hold me , feel me
Never end.

Like me, kiss me
set me free
Say you'd miss me

If I wasn't me.

Guard me, keep me
Safe from danger
Hug me, love me
Be no stranger.

I'm true, I'm real
Don't ignore me
I am, I feel
No tall story.

WHO THE HELL DO YOU THINK YOU ARE?

This one is all about how someone really made me angry by trying
to act all superior. As you can tell from reading this, it didn't go
down too well with me!

Who the hell do you think you are?
To pass judgement on me?
Your attitude is annoying me
You've pushed me way too far!

Sit there in your imagined eminence!
What you say bears no relevance
To what we are all debating!
You are just pontificating!

I feel my anger rising to it's peak
I think I'm going to explode!
I am so annoyed I cannot speak!
Malodorous little toad!

Give me a dragon's tongue of sharp steel
And I'll run it straight through you!
As you pay no heed to how I feel
Repellent through and through!

You just irritate me so damned much!
You're like German Measles
You really are so out of touch
Creeping little weasel!

So go away and let me be me
Don't speak to me again!
And I'll enjoy being so free
Without you oh psychic drain!

IS IT TRUE...?

A bit of fun.......!

One for sorrow, two for joy
That's how the saying goes
Is a girl worth less than a boy?
I guess we'll never know!

VIVE LA.....

Another 'hyper' poem!

Down with the monarchy!
Let's sample anarchy!
Forget the hierarchy!
Banish the patriarchy!

Vive la difference!
Goodbye to ignorance!
It has no significance!
Bring us some deliverance!

Get rid of arrogance!
Aristocratic dalliance!
Supposed elegance!
All smacks of negligence!

Power is relinquished!
Juvenile delinquents!
Is it just coincidence?
The awful consequence!

HURT...AGAIN

This is all about self-harm and how I used to do it – at the command of Mr Sarky, and how it made me feel ten times worse afterwards as not only was I upset, I was also in physical pain. It also includes my pledge never to do this again. I've not done it now for over 2 years!

Another wound-I'm hurt again
My arm weeps scarlet tears
Yet even though I feel the pain
It does not calm my fears.

Another wound-I'm hurt again
Can't speak for I'm struck dumb
Yet even though I feel the pain
My heart and soul are numb.

Another wound-I'm hurt again
My flesh is raw and torn
Yet even though I feel the pain
All I receive is scorn.

Another wound-I'm hurt again
I am in such a mess
Yet even though I feel the pain
I have just loneliness.

Another wound-I'm hurt again
And no-one ever knows
Yet even though I feel the pain
As my precious blood flows.

Another wound-I'm hurt again
Beneath a weeping willow
Yet even though I feel the pain
I sob into my pillow.

But...........?

Another wound?Stop!No more pain!
I've turned myself around

Tales from a Broken Mind

I'll never hurt myself again
For that I am so proud.

LIFE ON THE RAZOR'S EDGE

This one is all about winning the battle against self-harm.

I used to live my life
Upon the razor's edge
A sharply bladed knife
My skin to pain I pledged

I used to self destruct
On a daily basis
Until my life I plucked
Away from the pain-chasers.

I used to rip myself
Apart yet stayed together
'Twas not good for my health
Could not go on forever.

I used to be this girl
Who carved pain upon her skin
But now I see the world
As a place where I might win.

I used to feel so frightened
Alone and insecure
But now I am enlightened
I am petrified no more!

So please just look around you
Before you grab that knife
And you will see that it's true
You really can choose life.

SCAR(R)ED

Again, this one is all about self-harm and escaping it's ugly grip.

I'm scared, I'm scarred
An imperfection
Cut and bruised
I need protection.

I'm scared, I'm scarred
Heinous transgression
Hurt, and used
Raging incandescent.

I'm scared, I'm scarred
Yet worth no mention
Tired, confused
Need intervention.

I'm scared, I'm scarred
My flame extinguished
Dead, abused
My life relinquished.

I'm scared, I'm scarred
And treated horridly
wrongly accused
Of reacting floridly.

I'm scared, I'm scarred
But life goes onward
Yesterday's news?
No! I'm moving forward!

JUMBLED WORDS...

This is all about how my thoughts get a bit, well, jumbled at times!

I know just what I need to say
But my words are just a jumble
My confidence- it fades away
And my voice becomes a mumble.

I try to speak- you shoot me dead
You won't let me have my say
You tell me it's all inside my head
And you wish I'd go away.

You won't even give me a chance
Can't bear to hear my voice
I wish you'd change your biased stance
And let me have a choice.

Are you afraid of what I'll say?
Or do you just not want to listen?
You think that I'll just fade away
Don't see my tears that glisten.

For sticks and stones may break your bones
But my words they will not hurt you
Please step out of your comfort zones
And I'll tell how it is to you.

So please, I beg you - include me
Although my thoughts are jumbled
And when words do elude me
Don't panic-I just stumbled!

THIS SCARES ME......

This is all about how after a while without self-harming, I realised the potential danger I had put myself in and how scary that was for me. It's also about regrets as I now have permanent scarring to my left forearm that I will be stuck with for life. I guess I just have to learn to accept it, but it's hard to do that sometimes- especially when you know that it was you that did it to yourself.

The scars I etched on my own skin
Though nothing quite prepared me
To see the state that I was in
And this is just what scared me.

My best friend was a razor blade
Though nothing quite prepared me
To see the damage that I made
And this bloody well scared me.

I wish that I could turn back time
Though nothing quite prepared me
And from despair to hope I'd climb
And this was just what scared me.

I wounded myself so savagely
Though nothing quite prepared me
To see the scars that ravaged me
And this bloody well scared me.

DON'T DO IT!

This one is about trying to talk myself out of suicide.

You're feeling angry, upset, hurt
But please put down that knife
For it is never really worth
The ending of your life.

You're feeling dead behind the eyes
But please, put down that gun
Please don't write your last goodbyes
And snuff out the dying sun.

You're feeling awful, crazy, sad
But please put down those pills
For even when life feels so bad
Death never fulfils.

YOU DIDN'T CARE........

This is an anger poem that I wrote about all the people (and there
have been plenty of them), who wrote me off- mostly when I was an
adolescent and was first becoming unwell. I still hope they will read
this book and acknowledge that I am not the waste of space that
they seemed to think I was and that I proved them wrong.

I sat there and wanted to scream at you
For hurt inflicted way back then
But no! I am so much stronger than that
And I'd never trust you again.

You wrote me off and then tossed me aside
And it hurt me like bloody hell
Yet you couldn't even force a smile
Now I'm freed from that cell.

Well now I've got some news for you old pal!
I am gettin' along just fine
And it's with no thanks to you, you see
The impetus was all mine!

So go stick your opinions somewhere else
For it's no longer I will hear
'You have no therapeutic goals'
Your ignorance I'll not fear!

MOVIN' ON...

This is a poem all about moving on with my life and not taking on board all the horrible things that some people- mostly bullies, said or insinuated to me in the past.

You hurt me when you criticise
The things I say and do
I see the scorn within your eyes
Is that really you?

You hurt me when you give that look
For it's making me cry
For is not life an open book?
At least until we die?

You hurt me when you say those words
Do you know what they mean?
They're more than just nouns and verbs
They make me want to scream!

You hurt me when you do not hear
The things I need to say
As if I should just disappear
You want me thrown away.

You hurt me when you will not see
The person that's inside
One day you'll realise it's me
Will you still be so snide?

You hurt me when you knock me back
As though I mean nothing
But one day that veneer will crack
And I'll be the one laughing!

You hurt me so much in the past
Yet I am now the one
Who's getting back her life-and fast
Cos I am movin' on...

THESE FOUR WALLS

This poem is all about how I think in a somewhat sideways fashion
sometimes and how I come out with totally random ideas.

If these four walls could talk to me
I wonder what they'd say
What deep, dark secrets they'd impart
Or silent, sombre, grey.
And if they were to speak to me
would we have conversation?
Or would we just sit staring, still
And never get anywhere?
For walls have eyes and ears it's true
They witness everything
But never give up their solemn truths
So loyal are they to friends.
And who needs ceilings when you've got walls?
They are dull and lifeless!
And floors? Who wants to stay here, grounded
When we could float in ether?
The walls they are our confidantes
And in them we should trust
For they know all that has been said
But they never divulge a word......

DO WHATEVER

This is another anger poem that basically tells people who annoy me
where they can go!

Rip my heart out stamp on it!
Stick it in your pocket
If you want to then you can
Wear it as a locket!

Pinch me punch me-anything
You think you're so clever
Nothing really bothers me
So just go do whatever!

Love me, hate me-like I care!
Go on and do your worst!
I couldn't give damn mate!
You wouldn't be the first!

So now you stick your neck out
You think you're so damn hot
I've got some news for you
You're just so bloody NOT!

FUN?

This is an anger poem that allowed me to express how I feel about
the voices who try to put me down.

You seem to think that hurting me
Is just some kind of fun
But I won't take it personally
To me you are no-one!

You think you are "hip" and "cool"
It's just part of your fun
But I know you're a stuck-up fool
To me you are no-one!

You seem to think you own me
But you had better run
Your ignorance-you've shown me
To me you are no-one!

Your arrogance? I just laugh
Are you really that dumb?
Or are you havin' a giraffe?
To me you are no-one!

You try to patronise me
With words designed to stun
But I recognise, see
That you are just no-one.

THE 'ROOM'

This poem is all about undertaking therapy and exposing vulnerabilities.

The walls are closing in on me
The air is getting short
How is it that this simple room
Makes me feel like I'm caught?

It feels just like I am spinning
But I also feel trapped
What is it 'bout this simple room
Reflects me when I snapped.

I sit and pour my heart out
Sat within in that chair there
But something in this simple room
Makes my soul feel so bare.

WISHFUL THINKING......

This one is about feeling held back in terms of reaching my potential in a number of areas of my life. I suppose I am quite ambitious in some respects but with ambition come roadblocks - either people or situations that hold you back and stifle you. For most of my working life I have been in the 'assistant' role and it frustrates me. I know I am capable of so much more than the constraints of jobs allow me to do. I am doing a Psychology degree to help myself move forwards and hope that it leads me to what I really want.

I wish that I could float away
Out through the open windows
I wish that I could float away
Upon the breeze that blows

I need to get on out of here
Before my brain implodes
I need to get on out of here
In case it all explodes

I can't bear feeling trapped like this
Never reaching my potential
I can't bear feeling trapped like this
Is life just existential?

I know I can do things others can
But no-one seems to believe
I know I can do things others can
So why can't I achieve?

People always pass me over
Please, go on, just go ahead
Keep on passing me over
For ambition is now dead....

And was it real all the while?
Or is it just wishful thinking?
That people can't see through the smile

And see my heart is sinking.....?

AND THIS IS WHAT I SAW......

Another poem about extra-special life experiences...!!!

Psst! Listen to what I saw last night!
Some strange mythological creatures!
They didn't half give me a fright!
With their gnarled and wizened features!

Psst! Listen to what I saw last night!
Some peculiar men with no faces!
I checked to see if I was right,
And I saw just empty spaces!

Psst! Listen to what I saw last night!
Magical colours that bridged the void!
Now was something wrong with my sight?
I saw them- I'm not paranoid.

Psst! Listen to what I saw last night!
Such an amazing psychedelic sky!
Waiting for reality to bite
And I still don't know quite why!

Psst! Listen to what I saw last night!
An amazing carnival around my bed!
It was cool until you put me "right"
Said it was all just in my head.........

BEWITCHED!

This was written whilst I was thinking in about a million directions all at the same time...!!!

This tragic tale of a boy and a girl
Who knew nothing at all about this world
Into which they were unceremoniously hurled
Is it any wonder that their lives unfurled?

This young girl-look,see her heart is aching
Could it be sadness or just the pills she's taking?
Either way her sadness is just so heart-breaking
Life at it's end when it should be in the making.

Of course I became so very concerned
When I found out, when I learned
Exactly for what her poor heart yearned
A boy whose future had all but burned.

A tale of woe-what could be worse?
Of young love lost- of love so cursed
If only this life could be rehearsed
Then maybe bad luck could be reversed!

......And nothing at all could have prepared me
I admit- the whole damned thing scared me
This tragic story must be shared see
And that's just the start of what they dared me...

But there are no words in the world you can ever say
Nothing that could ever these fears allay
For tragedy like this will never go away
The best you can do is to hold the beast at bay.

And now I have so much fear inside my head
It creeps about like the eternal un-dead
And the rivers with blood run scarlet- red
The tragic lovers could not find a welcoming bed.

There was something different about this young girl

Tales from a Broken Mind

Put quite simply, she was not of this world
Her teeth were pretty but her lips, they curled
She didn't walk- she floated and twirled......

Her hair was long and somewhat feathery
Her eyes they glistened somehow cleverly
Yet for one so young her skin was leathery
And the tears from her eyes fell all too readily......

That poor boy was caught in this lover's trap
Some would say foolish or call him a sap
Yet this girl whom he thought had fallen in his lap
Was dangerous and so likely to just SNAP!

But onwards they went, for love perseveres
'Tis strange what it is to the heart that endears
Even when you know it'll all end in tears
But when one is in love, one has no fears.

And what of the hero of this tragic tale?
A picture please for words just fail!
Flew he always across hill and dale
All for the love of a twisted female!

And caught in her web-to escape? NEVER!
For she is too devious, she is too clever
If he tries to escape her, his head she'll sever!
A cruel twist of fate for such brave endeavour!

To fly the nest, one must jump from the tree
Or never enjoy what it is to fly free!
And always stay wond'ring what could life be?
He whispered, "If only I had courage just to be me"

Young boy be afraid, be very afraid
Beware your dalliance with this poisonous maid!
For heroes are created, they are not made
Do not your valour for your life trade!

And she watches him from her witch's perch

Whisp'ring death- "He left me in the lurch!"
Soon by the neck he'll swing from a birch
In the old graveyard by the stone-built church.

He is oblivious, he knows not how
His life was going to be snuffed out
By a vain and heartless cow
The curtain will fall upon his final bow!

And still he looks and hopes to find
I know 'tis said that love is blind!
Be careful as the path does unwind
Erase that girl clear from your mind!

So they all shouted warnings across the park
They echoed, rebounded around in the dark
Yet still she left her fiendish little mark
She may sting like a hornet but she sings like a lark!

Run boy, run it's not too late
For you can still escape your fate
And her nails like knives did glisten and grate
Get away, quick boy! Don't succumb to fate!

And all the while she watches and sits,
A cruel smile plays upon her lips
Watch out boy- before she flips!
As into unconsciousness he slips........

A BILLION.........

This one is about feeling incredibly alone and isolated from the rest
of the world but also very victimised. It is also about how the voices
play 'mind-games' at times. This has happened to me on numerous
occasions and it doesn't get any less annoying!

A billion shards of shattered glass
They pierce my wounded heart
As misfortune's web- it seems so vast
It's tearing me apart.

A billion blades- see them glisten
Heading straight towards me
Yet still nobody wants to listen
Everyone ignores me.

A billion fires that rage so wild
They char my silky skin
And still they treat me like I'm a child
Can't see what is within.

A billion fumes that rise in plumes
Pollute the perfect sky
And now my loneliness just resumes
Yet no-one wonders why.

A billion screams that rip the air
Yet nobody can hear
This experience I cannot share
A terrifying fear.

A billion cries lost in the dark
Makes me feel so frightened
And hopelessness has made it's mark
No-one is enlightened.

A billion arrows fired from bows
And burning bright with flames
Still I am the only one who knows

Someone is playing mind-games.

A billion bursts of truest laughter
Now fill my secret mind
It's all ok, it's no disaster
As happiness I will find.

PSYCH APPOINTMENT

This poem is a bit of fun really. It is meant to be read as a dialogue between a Psychiatrist and a patient. It's all very tongue-in-cheek!

Do you recall when life went crazy?
Sorry Doc, my memory's hazy!
When did you first hear the voices?
Err, not sure- 'cos I've always heard noises!
Do you feel guilty of any crime?
Oh yes Doctor! All of the time!
Do you experience changes in mood?
Yeah, sometimes it's bad, sometimes it's good!
Do you feel low? Do you feel high?
Yes! Down in the dumps or up in the sky!
Do you ever believe that life is unreal?
Oh yes- that's exactly how I often feel!
Do you feel that life is a great big muddle?
I feel like I live inside a glass bubble!
Voices?-Inside or outside of your head?
Both Doc-telling me I should be dead!
Are these voices you hear ever kind?
Yes-but mostly they torment my mind!
Do you see strange sights with your own eyes?
Yes-sometimes they take me by surprise!
Do you feel paranoid-is the world out to get you?
So you heard it too Doc? The conspiracy is true!
Do you ever feel slowed up in your speech or movement?
Oh. Yes. Doc. tor. There's. Room. For. Im. Prove. ment!
Have you lost interest in things you enjoyed?
Well I can't do sex and that makes me annoyed!
Do you smell or taste things that really aren't there?
Well I once ate an apple that tasted like a pear!
Do you ever feel someone is reading your mind?
There's not much to read Doc- speak as you find!
What about alcohol or illicit drugs?
I only use beer-to drown snails and slugs!
Do you feel you're a risk to others or yourself?
Me? I'm a hazard to everyone's health!
Ok now we're done do you have any questions,

anything I've missed or any suggestions?
So, tell me Doc- what's your diagnosis?
I'm afraid my dear, you have psychosis!

WHY...?

This is a poem about overstepped boundaries.

Why did you touch me when I said 'no'?
You didn't leave me when I said 'go'

You had no right to impose yourself
You really screwed up my mental health

Who the hell do you think you are?
You pushed the limits way too far

I'd like to kick you where it hurts
And cut up all your favourite shirts

You seemed to think that you could do
To me anything you wanted to

I'll show you the anger,grief and ire
That fills my tortured soul with fire

I want to make you feel my pain
So you'll never do it again

And some day you will really see
That you are less than nothing to me.

TO GRANNY.........

Another poem about my Grandmother.

Another star has crashed and burned
And fallen from the sky
No time now for lessons learned
Nor chance to wonder why
But time aplenty to sit and ponder
'bout how it all went wrong
The tortured mind begins to wander
The heart begins to long
And what becomes of the yearning soul?
That glows and burns like fire
All that's left is a gaping hole
That once embraced desire
For no longer will those merry tones
Fill the airless void around us
The wind, it cries, shrieks and moans
And only serves to confound us
Farewell sweet angel, o' dearest one
We will always remember you
Your time to leave us now has come
For God has plans for you
So when you see us left down here
In times of dreaded angst or pain
Say a prayer to dry our tears
Until we are together again.

JEWEL

This is a bit of a nonsense poem that I wrote whilst in a particularly
good mood.

The rain pours down
And people frown
Such inclement weather
Under brollies
Shopping trollies
Feeling none too clever

Sadly single
cannot mingle
They hate to be alone
No note to fall
Into their hall
Another dial-tone.

Estranged couple
Strife and trouble
No wish to intervene
Just nod and smile
Inch for a mile
If you know what I mean!

A filthy slob
A stuck-up snob
God forbid they meet-up
And if they do
Trouble will brew
Who will win the beat-up?

A country dance
Balletic prance
Whatever takes your fancy
A sad old man
In a white van
Reads about necromancy!

A wise old owl
A chimney cowl
That billows fumes and smoke
Don't like to pry
But wonder why
Life feels like a sick joke.

A broken heart
That falls apart
At slightest provocation
Just keep good time
And you'll be fine
Avoid procrastination!

Tormented mind
One day you'll find
Some kind of inner peace
It will come good
They said it would
Will wonders never cease?

So please stay cool
Enlightened fool
Don't let things get you down
For you're a star
You know you are
Another jewel in life's crown.

OTHER PEOPLE...

This is a poem about how I try not to internalise the stupid things others sometimes say to me. Let's face it -some people do say some daft things at times whether intentional or not. It is best to try and learn to let these stupid comments 'bounce' off you and not to pay too much attention to them.

People say 'you're mad, you're crazy'
But I don't really care!
Their stupid comments never faze me
To me they are not there!

Why do people think that they
Have the right to insult me?
I wish that they would go away
Their faces just revolt me!

And to their damned, ridiculous lies
I will never listen
They will never make me cry
Nor cause sad tears to glisten!

Why do people point and stare
And mock my every move?
I am me- just plain ol' Claire
I have nothing to prove!

So they can stick their stupid words
Where the sun don't shine!
For they're the ones who are absurd
And me? I am just fine!

FACES.........

This is about how seeing the faces of the people I love, calms me.

Anger burning deep inside
Swelling like a rising tide

Overwhelmed by dejection
Solitude like an infection

Hatred that consumes the soul
Hearts will stop, heads will roll

Fear and loathing in the brain
Feel the awful crushing pain

Scared, hurt, shocked and frightened
But never, ever feel enlightened

Uncontrollable emotion
Feels as mighty as the ocean

Hate feeds hate and fear feeds fear
Hold me closer, hold me near

The walls are closing in too tight
Come, get me out , save me tonight

I feel like I've just hit the ceiling
No longer quite sure how I'm feeling

But every time I see your face
I smile 'cos you're my saving grace.

OAK TREE

This is all about disrespect and wanton destruction of life's natural beauty.

There used to be an old oak tree
That stood proud in a field
But that was when the land was free
Before they started to build.

They took a chainsaw to it's trunk
And cackled as it fell
Tossed aside like some old junk
Timber! Was the oak's death knell.

Massacred it lay dismembered
Strewn 'cross the cold, wet ground
It will always be remembered
As 'neath it, solace was found.

To butcher it was a great crime
To kill such majesty
For I recall a much happier time
Before this travesty.

I used to sit beneath it's boughs
Breeze whisp'ring through it's leaves
And watch contented sheep and cows
Until it's life was thieved.

Now there stands a housing estate
Where once that great tree stood
To save this tree it is too late
Reduced to firewood.

Another soulless tenement
imposing on our sight
Ubiquitous development
We lost to you our fight.

NUTS!

Another nonsense poem......

All this madness all around
It surely must be catching
All the ideas to be found
Crazy dreams a-hatching!

Round the twist or round the bend
Just call it what you want to
Insanity is my best friend
Ignore all those that taunt you.

As nutty as a fruitcake
Or mad as a march hare
All the comments that they make
Me? I just don't care!

But madness- it surrounds us
I see it crystal clear
It's there- it's all around us
There is no need to fear!

So go ahead- be free now
Go let your madness out
Get crazy any old how
Dance and sing and shout!

THE GIFT

An uplifting poem about the good parts of life. Having a mental health problem does not mean that life can never be enjoyable or fulfilling. I think we have to be grateful for our time on earth and make good use of it. Life's too short to be negative all of the time.

Hopes and dreams are precious things
At least that's what I've found
They are what keep us alive
'Til we're six feet 'neath the ground!

Treasure every moment here
Upon this fragile earth
Life's too short to harbour fear
Though death precedes rebirth.

Be kind to your fellow man
We're all created equal
When life doesn't go to plan
We can't just write the sequel!

We have one life, just one chance
Let's try to have some fun
We should sing, we should dance
Underneath the golden sun.

So don't sit there and waste your life
Pondering the what-ifs
No more struggle, no more strife
Enjoy this precious gift!

Claire Attwood

NO MORE........

This poem is all about how I beat self-harm (and the voices) and
will never do it again.

No more pain will I inflict
Upon my own soft skin
For I have won my conflict
I thought I'd never win.

No more will I live my life
Upon the razor's edge
For I'll no longer deal with strife
By causing myself damage

No more will I feel that urge
To see my own blood flow
Nor feel the need to cleanse or purge
I've moved on and let go!

No more will I sense the need
To hurt me 'cos of others
I don't have to see me bleed
To get rid of my bothers.

No more will I see a knife
And feel that grim temptation
For I have recovered my life
And it's a great sensation!

No more will I self-chastise
Nor blame myself for bad luck
For life has opened up my eyes
And I'm no longer stuck!

TALES FROM A BROKEN MIND

This is about how it is possible to move on from the experience of mental ill-health.

All these stories here you'll find
Are but tales from a broken mind

All true stories of love, of hate
How I escaped a cruel fate

Some despair, some devotion
Never devoid of raw emotion

Just as the tide governs the sea
So my broken mind has set me free

Happiness? I have one suggestion
Don't be afraid to challenge and question

Life is hard but you will cope
Just stay focussed and don't give up hope

Try to keep things in perspective
Keep it real and be objective.

If you can do all of this
You may just find life is bliss!

THE VOICES THAT I HEAR

This is about feeling that I will never be free of Mr Sarky's
negativity. He has been with me for as long as I can remember and I
truly believe he will remain with me for the rest of my life.
However- I would like to get to a point where I am more in charge
and don't have to put up with all his nonsense!

You're worthless, you're trouble-
They shout when they torment my ears
Reduce my self-esteem to rubble
The voices that I hear.

They're always there, where e'er I go
And they are always bad
I feel like screaming NO, NO, NO!
But people would think I'm mad!

They're there to torture my sick brain
Drop poison in my mind
Sometimes I feel ill with the pain
No solace can I find.

They follow me everywhere it's true
They're always at my shoulder
It doesn't matter what I do
Their breath is getting colder.

I feel them breathing on my skin
I wish they'd leave me alone
It feels like I'll never win
This battle of my own.

They make their eerie presence known
Almost every hour
And yet they've not quite shown
The extent of their power.

Sometimes it's just Mr Sarky
Sometimes it's a crowd
Always the same old malarkey

Tales from a Broken Mind

Starts off quiet, ends up loud.

I wonder if I'll ever be free
From their vile grip
I will keep on being me
Though they won't let their masks slip......

THEATRE OF LIFE............

This is a poem about something I feel when I am unwell. I often consider that maybe life isn't real and that we are all just actors in a huge play.

Life is an elaborate game
That we can never win
Sometimes laughter, sometimes shame
Full of virtue, full of sin.

Life's not real, it's too absurd
To be completely true
Transient like the spoken word
A bit of a to-do!

We are all actors in a play
Come on- take centre stage!
For all we have at the end of the day
A guilty conscience to assuage!

Jack be nimble, Jack be quick
Just don't hang 'round too long
For Jack found out that life is sick
Please don't sell out your soul!

The curtain closes on the last night
All stars come take your bows
Encores are over, out of sight
Is it real? Who cares anyhow!

The theatre's closed now, derelict
All that's left there are ghosts
That place where life was so damned slick
No glory now it boasts.

So spare a thought as you pass by
For life has run it's course
It's so sad, it'll make you cry
Walking past it's abandoned doors.

Tales from a Broken Mind

No more laughter, no more joy
Resounds around it's walls
Goodbye to all the girls and boys
As the final curtain falls.

For as I said before to thee
Life's a complex angst-ridden hoax
My words were true and now you see
That life is just a joke!

MANIC!

A hyper poem!

The craziness is ever-present
My blood is fizzing- effervescent!
Rushing round, I'm always busy
Sometimes I make myself feel dizzy!

I'm bouncing here, there, everywhere
Driving myself to the point of despair!
I can't slow down, nor stop and rest
I don't know what to do for the best!

It's crazy, nuts and totally manic
My heart it races like I'm in a panic!
You'd think I'd be tired but I'm not
That's how much energy I've got!

I'm practically bouncing off the walls
I'm breaking all of gravity's rules!
On the ground, then up in the air
Doing whatever- I don't care!

All my blood's around me pumping
Gives me the strength to keep on jumping!
Up and down and round and round
My feet don't even touch the ground!

Okay- now I feel like I'm fit to drop
But still my racing mind won't stop!
I'm worn out now, I am so tired
I need my brain to be rewired!

So now I will just try to chill
Calm it down 'cos I feel ill!
I wish that I could have a rest
'Cos being hyper is such a pest!

Tales from a Broken Mind

MY CELL...........

This is fairly self-explanatory. Basically it is about how feeling
mentally unwell can feel like being imprisoned but also how
recovery can make you feel free again.

Sometimes when I am feeling unwell
It's just like being in a prison cell.
Heavy steel door, bars at the window
Gripped by fear that won't let me go.

I guess this is just my consignment
Abandoned in solitary confinement
Half an hour in the prison yard
Breaking rocks is oh so hard.

Hoping everyday for that elusive pardon
All I ever see is a miserable warden
I wish I could escape and be so free
'Cos these walls are closing in on me!

I pray to have a glimpse of the stars
Without peering out from behind bars
I long to hear the birds and bees
And enjoy the summer breeze.

My only company is the voices
Not the best of all life's choices
All I get is strange, weird visions
And still I feel like I'm in prison.

So Mr Sarky- leave me alone
Let me out- I long for home
In my cell I had no fun
But now I'm free and on the run!

I WISH I WAS SOMEONE ELSE...

I think we have all been in this place before-wishing we were
someone else. But as everyone has problems, I guess we'd just have
different problems. Maybe that's the attraction...!

If only things were different
And maybe I had a choice
I wish I was someone else
Someone who has a voice.

It feels so dis-empowering
At the mercy of my mood
I wish I was someone else
Someone who is good.

I want to be successful
To win once in a while
I wish I was someone else
Someone who can smile.

If only people could see
The hurt I have inside
I wish I was someone else
Someone who feels pride.

I wish I didn't hate myself
I wish I could be free
I wish I was someone else
Someone but not me.

People see the outside
And not what is within
I wish I was someone else
Someone who can win.

I wish that people saw past
The mask I always wear
I wish I was someone else
Anyone but Claire.

WHAT THEY SAID..........

This is another poem about voice hearing and how unkind voices
can be. It does feel like I am the victim of some great conspiracy
sometimes and Mr Sarky is the ring-leader-no surprises there then...!

Look at her- stupid cow!
That is what they said
Let's go ruin it now
She'll soon wish she was dead!

Ha ha ha! She's so unwise!
That is what they said
Let's fool her ears- and her eyes!
Laughed the voices round my head.

See her there- ah! She's crying!
That is what they said
'Cos she knows we are spying
And won't leave her 'til she's dead!

Everyone knows she's a freak
That is what they said
For she hears every word we speak
The voices by her head.

See what we can do to her?
That is what they said
We can turn her day sour
Make her mind feel dead!

We can reduce her to tears
That is what they said
Bring to life all her fears
Say the voices round my head.

BLEAK...

The wild and wily west wind wails
Across the bleak cold moor
Solitary, sad the solemn ship sails
Yet no-one knows what for.

Battered, beaten, broken blooms
Of lonely dying flowers
Lingering, languishing, large it looms
In just a matter of hours.

EXCLUDED...

This is all about how I used to feel in the sixth form common room at school- on the rare occasions I dared to go in there. I don't think that there is anything more isolating than feeling alone whilst surrounded by other people. It really drives it home to you that no-one likes you and that you are excluded. I was bullied all the way through high school and half of middle school. If I ever hear anyone say that being bullied is 'character-building', I think I will lose the plot! It isn't character building at all- it is hideous, vile and soul-destroying.

I'm sitting in a crowded room
With people all around me.
They're talking, whispering, laughing
And I am not a part of it.
The conversations stop and start

The pitch rises and falls
The volume seems to fluctuate
But I am not a part of it
So why should I even care?
I try my hardest to join in
But no-one heeds my voice
It's like I am invisible
As I am not a part of it.
I am a survivor
I came through difficult times
I wish you all could see this
Yet I'm not a part of it.
It feels like I'm not there
Like somehow I'm excluded
Everybody else is heard
But I am not a part of it.
I may have a troubled past
But it's only made me stronger
So please don't treat me differently
Like I'm not a part of it.

PARANOIA

This one is all about how it feels to experience paranoia and how it infiltrates every aspect of your life.

Paranoia.
Such a horrid little word.
Paranoia.
Twisted everything I heard.
Paranoia.
So damned ubiquitous.
Paranoia.
Makes me so suspicious.
Paranoia.
Influences all my thoughts.
Paranoia.
A whisper and I'm caught.
Paranoia.
Like a knife in my back.
Paranoia.
My mind starts to crack.
Paranoia.
Won't leave me alone.
Paranoia.
Wherever I go.
Paranoia.
I beg you to free me.
Paranoia.
But no-one believes me.
Paranoia...................

BE GONE.....

This is a very angry poem that I wrote in sheer temper after Mr
Sarky really annoyed and upset me. I am not usually an angry
person- but I refuse to be spoken to or treated the way this voice did
to me. Usually I am fairly placid!

Ok so now you've really blown it.
I can't take this bullshit any more.
I'm sick and tired of you
So now I'm showing you the door.

Take back every vicious word
Every poisonous little lie
Stick your knife elsewhere
Watch your power slowly die.

If you think you're coming back
You'd better think again
Your words are too destructive
They fall like acid rain.

And me? I don't care for you
Like you never cared for me
You only looked after number one
News flash! Now I'm free!

So walk away now I'll not worry
In fact I couldn't care less.
When you're gone from my life
I'll finally feel my best.

LEAVE ME ALONE

This is about how sometimes other people think that they know best
and that they have the right to take over and do things 'for' me when
I am actually quite capable of doing things for myself- I just do
them in my own little way.

Leave me alone, please go away
If I wanted your help I'd ask
It's my life and I have final say
So relieve yourself of your task.

I am more than fit and able
To say what I want to say
I will lay my cards on the table
So leave it and go away!

You've no right telling me what to do
Towards you I feel myself souring,
You treated me like a child of two
Totally dis-empowering!

BRAIN TANGLE...

This is about how I become somewhat chaotic and my brain feels all
tangled up. My thoughts whizz around in all directions and I need
space to try and get my head back together. Mr Sarky doesn't like to
give me a break though and always adds to the confusion. This
really annoys me!

Everybody go away!
Please don't bug me, not today
I need time and I need space
Would you get out of my face?

I've got things I have to do
You've got free time? Lucky you!
Please stop going on and on
Now my concentration's gone.

Jabber, jabber on at me
I am busy-can't you see?
I just have to draw the line
If it's urgent-we'll talk at nine.

Look inside my muddled head
Question marks and tangled thread
Silent forces, watching me
I will never again be free.

My mind's spotlight is going dim
And all my ideas start to swim.
I try to recover what I once had
But it's all gone now and I feel sad.

On the outside I look alright
But no one sees the tears at night.
It's all because I'm feeling low
I'm scared to let my anguish show.

IF I COULD ONLY......

This is all about how tempting it feels to just give up rather than keep struggling. But it also suggests that it won't necessarily solve anything.

If I could only flick the switch
Turn the lights out cos life's a bitch
I am sure it would be okay
One less nuisance in their way
But things are never cut and dried
Even in death by suicide!

If I could only seize the day
Just do it right and fade away
I'd be gone, they'd close the curtain
It would suit them for certain
But who knows where our fate will land
Even in death by one's own hand!

If I could only find the strength
I've thought about this plan at length
And no more will I interfere
Hear them laugh and hear them cheer
But they'll lie that 'we never heard her'
Even in death by self-murder.

DEPRESSION............

This short poem simply describes how depression makes everything
seem bleak and hopeless.

Depressing, darkened, hidden thoughts
Plough through my mind like juggernauts.

Turn all my dreams into black knights
Hidden in my mind- out of sight.

Poisonous- a vicious rumour
Stealing laughter, stealing humour.

WHAT IF.....

This was written when I was happy but also feeling very paranoid
about things.

What if a kiss
From my sweet lover's lips
Was just a kiss
And not a taste of impending doom
Of a life not worth living
Of unending gloom?
What if that moment
As sacred as my soul
Was just for one minute
A glimmer of hope, a ray of light
Not about death
But of wonder and life?
What if those words
That are spoken are true
That really mean something
And not hollow lies
Or a million goodbyes?
What if the embrace
That I unfurl myself into
Was pure, innocent love
And nothing more sinister
Or a final gesture?
What if I could see
With hope-filled eyes
Instead of these clouds
Which hang over me?
If I could just for one moment
Be freed from this spell
These chains that bind me
In bitterest hell.
And sample the beauty
The depth of wonder
And for that precious minute
Just know, just know

That everything is all right

Then maybe I could let go
And not slip into free fall
But taste one sweet drop
Of life's sweet elixir
From an un-poisoned chalice
And float for a while
See angels and cherubs
And feel I belong
Just for one moment.
What if..................?

SHADOW...

This is all about visual hallucinations.

It's there- it's there
I saw it - I swear!
It seems to follow me
Everywhere!
If I run-it runs
If I stop- it stops
Turn left- turn right
Try as I might
It's a darkened
Copy of me!
Of it I can't be free!
It's there all the time!
It never makes a sound
But I see it there!
Err wait a moment...
It's your shadow Claire!

Tales from a Broken Mind

YOU...........

This one is about Mr Sarky and illustrates how I battle with him.
This sort of battle occurs on almost a daily basis but is well worth
fighting as I find it empowering when I win!

You chase me through the morning
And hurry me through the night
And I know your intentions
Are driven by pure spite.

You might think you've got me fooled
Ha ha ha! That's just not so!
I see me in the mirror
And not your evil glow!

So be gone wooden faced one
Your power is diminished
I don't want you, just go
Your time is now finished!

BANANAS........

This is all about how I do what I call 'thinking sideways'. Thinking sideways happens when I distort what people have said/are saying to me. I think about the words they use and find alternative meanings in those words or take them very literally and it completely changes the message that the person is trying to convey! This can be quite entertaining at times but- it can also be a nuisance as I can't control it.

Some would say I've gone bananas
But that just makes me hoot
Cos why on earth would anyone
Look like a yellow fruit?

And they might say I've lost the plot
But what's that really worth?
Do they mean the story
Or a patch of earth?

They may say that I've gone crazy
 I don't really think so.
Do they know anything?
My guess would be 'No'.

Yet still they think that I am odd
Well here's something new-
I am perfectly sane
The one who's mad ...is you!

Tales from a Broken Mind

DRUNK...........

This one is fairly self-explanatory as it is all about feeling drunk and
out of control. I don't actually like the feeling of being drunk and
rarely drink alcohol.

I sit and ponder as the clouds drift by
About the wonder of blue skies.
For everything seems so much better
When we have some sunny weather.

Curiously strange and somewhat odd
I sit here and I pray to God.
Does it ever rain in Heaven
And do the shops shut at eleven?

I lay here and I start to think
I'm sober-give me some more drink!
Things start to become hazy
Am I drunk? Or just plain lazy?

I am unsure- is it the wine?
Cos an hour ago I was fine
But now my head starts to swim
And all my senses have gone dim!

I thought life was all full throttle
'Twas before I downed this bottle
Now I'm sure I'm not winning
I feel sick, the room is spinning

Those intelligent conversations
Now just feel like irritations
My body isn't mine now
I don't feel so good-ow!

My head is pounding I feel sick
Got so drunk, did it do the trick?
Nope. Now I feel rotten
By morning I'll have forgotten....

GIVE ME A BREAK.....

This is about Mr Sarky again and how I fight him when I am having a good day. I do get incredibly angry with him at times as he is very annoying and upsetting. I often swear at him to make him go away-it sometimes works but I have to be mindful of where I am at the time as it could be embarrassing if I did this in the middle of the supermarket!!!

Give what you give
And take what you take
But for pity's sake
Just give me a break!

Take the piss now
Just do whatever
I don't like you
And you're not clever.

In my ear hmm
I am not list'ning
You can shout yeah
I keep whistling!

Say your worst then
Go on say it now
I aint bothered
You're not so wow!

Givin' it this
Givin' it that
Do you know what?
You're such a prat!

So leave me alone
Cos I don't care
Go find someone
Else to scare!

THESE DAYS

This is about the way the media tend to focus on the bad things in life and how we should try to see beyond the gloomy side of life and enjoy the nicer aspects of it. It is so easy to become miserable or even depressed when we look at what the world's news is. The media often focus on the negative side of life-there must be a demand for it as people buy the papers etc.........

Times are hard it must be true
Cos I saw it on the news.
The papers all proclaim their doom
And perpetuate impending gloom.

We had the boom and now the bust
Institutions turning to dust!
This is what we hear every day
Depressing and scary all the way.

No one seems to want to laugh now
But we've got to rise somehow.
Lift your heads above all the ghosts
Come and raise your glasses to mine host!

For though the world may be losing
We can still do the choosing
So grit your teeth and practise your smile
For you all might need to for a while!

COLD.........

Another poem referring to Mr Sarky and his unpleasant personality.

Your eyes are cold
Your heart is hard
You do not care
It is unfair.

You have no soul
You like control
You are evil
Nasty weasel!

Your stare is dead
Your own sick head
You love the rain
And mock my pain.

Will you please leave
I don't believe
Your wicked tales
Love to deceive.

HOW CAN I EVER.....

This is a poem that I wrote when I was feeling particularly negative about life. Sometimes the recovery journey that we travel is not an easy one and there will be days when one feels like giving up. But it is worth the fight when you start to have more good days than bad days. Never give up.

How can I ever
Repair these broken wings?
Give them back their freedom?
Release them from bad dreams?

How can I ever
Free this captured soul?
Restore it to glory?
Away from this black hole?

How can I ever
Recover my own life?
Get back to the good times?
Free from this war and strife?

How can I ever
Walk toward the light?
When dark is all I see?
How can I get it right?

How can I ever
Begin to take a look?
Rediscover my life?
When it is a closed book?

KEEP IT TO YOURSELF........

This poem is all about how sometimes when I feel a little bit fragile,
I find it difficult to deal with other people being negative as it can
make me feel worse.

If you're bringing bad news
Please keep it to yourself.
For I can't handle any more
It harms my mental health!

If you are negative
Please just keep away
For I don't do sad stuff now
My nerves begin to fray!

If you're bringing tears
Please don't tell me
For I can't cry for you now
My eyes refuse to see!

STRONGER......

This poem is all about how other people let me down even though I was very supportive of them when they had problems. It is all about how I used to allow myself to be used as a doormat and how I refuse to be one any more!

For all those times I've sat and cried
Those endless hours I sacrificed.
For all the tears I've had to shed
Those bloody wounds that hurt and bled.
For all the nights I've laid awake
Those lonely times for my own sake.
For all the times I held that knife
Those urges to just end my life.
For all those times I sat and wondered
Those feelings burnt, lost and squandered.
For all the times I wanted out
Those days consumed with my self-doubt.
For all those times that were wasted
Those bitter lessons I have tasted.
For all those times I have been there
Those times I helped-but what would you care?
For all those times I mopped up your tears
Those times of sadness across all these years.
For all that friendship- what did I gain?
Those feelings of 'used' all over again.
But I'll not be your doormat much longer
I'm toughening up 'cos I am stronger.

FIGHTER...

I wrote this one when I was feeling more than somewhat paranoid
about life and about other people's intentions/motives. I was feeling
persecuted at the time-largely due to Mr Sarky and also because I
was feeling depressed.

I wish people could see
And understand
What it's like to be me
And halt the plan.

They've ignored my feelings
Unfortunate
With their wicked dealings
Discriminate!

Is it worth the struggle?
Embattlement
All these things to juggle?
Cold resentment.

With hearts hard and bitter
So judgemental
Their conscience like litter
Coincidental?

And their dark, evil eyes
Pure derision
As they spin webs of lies
Indecision.

As they sit and marvel
At their evil deeds
With skin cold as marble
Strangling weeds!

But I'll not be broken
Disfigurement
By evil words spoken
Embitterment!

For all their detritus
Eradicate
As they are not fighters
Exterminate!

My soul is much stronger
And infinite
For I'll battle longer
That's definite!

OPTIMIST/PESSIMIST...

This is about how when depressed I can be very pessimistic about life. Tip- try to be optimistic- or at least, realistic, as you will get so much more out of life.

For you there's a silver lining to every cloud
But I'm torn and tattered, decaying in a shroud.

For you there's joy when you wake in the morning
But I'm held back by a stark and bitter warning.

For you the world's a wonderful and happy place
But I have to fight to paint a smile on my face.

For you people listen, respect and value you
But I'm passed over, ignored with no real view.

For you you're a part of it, you're one of the team
But I'm on the outside- all I can do is dream.

For you the garden's rosy- always in full bloom
But all I see are strangling weeds, symbols of gloom.

For you the glass is always half full, always good
But my glass is half empty, can't see trees for wood.

For you are an optimist, you see the good side
But I am a pessimist swimming against the tide.

THE HATED...

This one is all about feeling unpopular.

Toll the old church bell
Tear the skies asunder
Throw me in the well
Then hold my head under!

Switch on the fountain
Rip the sun from the sky
Throw me off a mountain
And see if I can fly!

Stop! Hold the front page!
Blow the moon clean away
Trap me in a small cage
Get rid of me today!

Open the town hall
Because I guess you won
You watched my tragic fall
It's too late now I'm gone...

WHERE WERE YOU...?

This one refers to when I was 23 and I sought help for the first time.
Certain people who should have been there for me seemed to vanish
like snow in the sun! There is nothing like mental health problems
for showing you who your true friends are!

Where were you the day I fell apart?
The day it all went wrong
The day that all this did start?

Where were you when I needed you?
The time I lay in tears?
The time you should've been true?

Where were you when I was broken?
The moment I reached out?
The moment you should've spoken?

Where were you? I'll tell you for sure-
Walking away as I lay on the floor
Couldn't get fast enough out of the door
My obvious distress that you ignored.

I was always there for you
No matter what-I stood by you
As friends should- I loved you
But you only cared about YOU.

So now I cross that old street
Hoping so much that we don't meet
For I'd give a slap no kiss on the cheek
You're trash, you're sick, you're cheap!

THE DAY...

An optimistic little poem!

The day will come
I know for sure
When I will win
So don't ignore!

I have my plans
Be sure I do
And I will win
One over you!

Nothing stops me
I'm no flower
Cos I will win
Break your power!

I have thoughts
I have ideas
And I will win
Others have fears!

Be careful
How you treat me
Cos I will win
You won't beat me!

So caution!
Take great care
Cos I will win
Just you beware!

ONE SWEET DAY...

This one's just a bit of fun and was written when I was in quite a
silly mood!

One sweet day
I think 'twas early June
My snake and I
Went swimming on the moon.
We splashed around
But stayed bone dry
Hopped in a car
And started to fly

Along the way
We met a spider
A super-duper scooter rider
She spun her web of purest silk
Akin to most creatures of her ilk
She jumped in our car
And gave us directions
To a most bizarre interplanetary connection!

A tad far fetched?
I beg to differ for in that desert ran a river
The sun so hot we all did shiver
Our picnic was absolutely wizard
Well knock me down- there's my lizard!
She climbed aboard our little car
And promptly stated- ' To Mars!'
Well I'm not one to argue but....

On that sweet day I must just stress
I was not looking to digress
I had my plans all set in jelly
But left them underneath my telly!
So I had to take a sharp turn
At the intersection
At least my snake has a good sense of direction!
From him I will surely learn!

Tales from a Broken Mind

Round the corner we met a fish
So damned handsome-what a dish!
His golden fins
Caused my spider to spin
A web of purest golden sun
If only he knew what he'd begun!
This fish he told me to turn right
Ate my sat-nav with just one bite!

My snake and I were getting tired
All these passengers that we'd hired
All we wanted was a quiet swim
Keeps you fit like the gym
Instead we just got lost in space
Now would you all get out of my face!
Landing safely back on earth
A million cavies had given birth!

So we scarpered off my snake and I
And vowed never again in space to fly
We had our favourite conversation
All about wildlife conservation
But if you go for a swim on the moon
If you wish to I'll presume
Just be warned the flight leaves soon
And avoid the interplanetary loons!

LIES.........

This is all about the Government and how I don't trust politicians as
a rule!

Government lies, whips and spin
Politicians to truth are strangers
All around us peddling sin
We all must wise up to the dangers.

They feed us on foul falsehoods
And obnoxiously reel us all in
Fail to deliver the goods
Pseudo-democracy wearing thin!

Insincere, promise broken
This dishonourable collection
Lie after lie is spoken
Seems we all made the wrong selection!

For politicians tell lies
Whilst the rest of us seek for the truth
You can see it in their eyes
The incontrovertible proof!

So beware the politician
For he has made telling lies an art
All of his own volition
From a blackened and twisted heart.

ME. I. MYSELF...

This is all about feeling divided.

Which one of me will you hurt today?
Me, I or Myself?
I try to protect all three you see
To maintain some kind of health.

For my Me is somewhat fragile
Just like cracking ice
And although I may attempt to smile
Please-can't you just be nice?

My I? It's rather delicate
Just like a flower
Oh, and just because you think like that
Does not give you power!

Myself? I am not in great health
What you see is me
But I do not envy you your stealth
Because at least I'm free!

PAIN.........

This is all about how mental health problems make people feel so low- especially when there is a lack of adequate support...

Pain, pain
Falls like rain
Swirling flash flood in the gutter
Leave her- just another nutter
She's cracked up again.

When, when
Please my friend
Watch her crawl upon her knees now
Oh just ignore her anyhow
She went mad just then.

Why, why
Does she cry
For distant dreams so far away
She clings to life day by day
Insane, silent sigh.

Tears, tears
All her fears
The terrors that rip her apart
Hidden deep within her heart
No-one dares draw near.

Turn, turn
Will she learn
That truly no-one wants to know
They all wish that she'd just go
No more their concern...

DOSED...........

This is one I wrote when I was fed up with taking meds and got a bit
stroppy about it all!

Pop a pill
To cure your ill
Take your fill
Oh, here's the bill.

I am dosed
My brain is toast
I won't boast
Oh, make the most.

Take the meds
To clear your head
Don't stay in bed
Oh, should have said.

I am dosed
Is this supposed
To clear the coast
Oh, brain cells roast.

Co-operate
Procrastinate?
Not worth the wait
Oh, filled with hate.

I am dosed
Chemical host
Tied to a post
Oh, sicker than most...

ANSWERS?...

This is all about how people who think they know best try to explain away the experiences that I have.

You question my stubbornness
My strong defiance
Cos what I experience
Aint explained by science

You question my attitude
My thoughts do not yield
Cos what I experience
Explains how I feel

You question my abilities
My will to succeed
But what I experience
Explains what I need

You question my agony
My 'wrongly wired' brain
But what I experience
Explains all my pain

You question my chemistry
My 'synaptic junk'
But what I experience
Explains why I've sunk

You question my solitude
Don't like how I'm alone
But what I experience
Explains just how I've grown.

GO!...........

This is another one about feeling excluded by my peer group-mostly relating to when I was at school. Oh happy days...NOT!!!

Go! Enjoy your parties
Quickly, girls go on
Just don't look o'er your shoulders
For me cos I'll be gone.

Go! Enjoy your young lives
Before it's too late
Just don't look into the past
For me it is too late.

Go! Enjoy your freedom
As long as it lasts
Just don't gaze on backwards
For me it went too fast.

SPARE ME...........

This one is about wishing I didn't feel the way I often do and of
wanting someone to take it all away.

Take from me this veil of darkness
This sorry shroud of deepest black
And light the path of sombre sadness
Guide me on my journey back.

Smash these rocks that do so hinder
These thistles that pierce my pale skin
Release me from this harsh, cruel winter
Before the ice becomes too thin.

Make for me these spindly trees fall
Destroy their gnarled boughs and branches
Support me as I stagger and crawl
Through the flick'ring fire that dances.

Take from me these Hellish visions
These voices that shatter the silence
Save me from this damned derision
This life of pain and violence.

Remove from me these blackened feelings
Save me from this cruel twist of fate
Protect me from their evil dealings
Help me before it is too late.

LIGHT IN HER EYES..........

This one was written when I felt depressed and felt I didn't have the strength to go on.

Look at that girl there
The light has gone from her eyes
But if you really knew her
You wouldn't be so surprised.

You see, that girl there
She never asked for too much
And if you really knew her
You would long to feel her touch.

Because that girl there
She had a heart of gold
And if you really knew her
You would never feel the cold.

The light behind her eyes
It seems it burned too bright
So look up to the skies
For she's a star tonight.

NASTY...........

A poem about how scary it is when I experience what I call 'waking dreams'. In these dreams it feels as though I am awake and that whatever horrible dream I am having, is reality.

Save me from this sneaking slumber
That masquerades as sweetest sleep
And stop me now from falling under
It's subtle spell my soul to keep

The breath of darkness creepily
Lays it's shadow across my face
I feel a scream rise deep in me
But it's vanished without a trace.

Pull me from this waking horror
This acrid, foul, repellent stench
Smash up every glass and mirror
And help me stop it's vile revenge.

SEASIDE SUICIDE!

This is about how one of the voices I hear, Mr Sarky, tries to
ambush me at every given possibility to make me feel bad.

I see the sea
Keep walking, keep walking
It's tempting me
Ignore it, ignore it
Want to jump in
Resist it, resist it
Oblivion
Keep fighting, keep fighting
Pulling me close
Step back now, step back now
Mind overdosed
Be strong now, be strong now
Constant battles
Just stop it, just stop it
Sick mind rattles
Come on now, come on now
Slipping under
Don't think that, don't think that
Cold sea thunder
Reach out now, reach out now
Strong undertow
Come back now, come back now
Time to let go
Grab my hand, grab my hand
Verdict? Insane!
Gone mad now, gone mad now
A losing game
Too late now, too late now...........

BATHROOM SORROW

This is another one about crying alone at night and also about my
promise never to harm myself again because of the voices I hear.

Little crumpled heap
Upon the bathroom floor
They all try to sleep
But I cry more and more.

Beneath the basin
Feeling all that sorrow
My heart is racing
Thinking of tomorrow.

A pathetic sight
Behind the bathroom door
Will it be tonight?
My open wounds are raw.

Looking at a blade
Upon the bathroom shelf
A promise I made
A deal made with myself.

And as my tears fall
Onto the bathroom tiles
All I do is crawl
Along what seems like miles.

Should I reach for it?
That simple solution?
No! I don't want it
Made a resolution.

My healed wound meshes
No more tears to be wept
For there is nought so precious
As a promise kept.

THE LIAR HERE.............

This is one about Mr Sarky and his lies.

The endless searching of the soul
To find that inner mysticism
Feelings that are out of control
Ravaged by cruellest criticism.

You say I should remain grounded
Exercise good old realism
But your fears are unfounded
Tied up in your selfish narcissism.

You tell stories that just aren't true
Blame it all on my cynicism
But the liar here is you
With your wicked, nasty pessimism.

So be gone you creep-out of my ears
And take your evil fatalism
You're worth no more of my tears
Cos my new life's breathing optimism!

HAVE FUN AT MY EXPENSE.......

This is all about being the object of ridicule.

If it's laughter
That you're after
Go ahead and mock me
I don't mind
If you're unkind
I'm used to it you see.

And ridicule
So very cruel
If that is what you're seeking
Then make fun
In front of everyone
Heckle me when I'm speaking.

If it's proof
Of the truth
Or searching for clarity
Do as you please
And don't mind me
I've lost my sanity!

SHUT UP!

This is all about how sometimes, things that have no personal
relevance to me, seem to take on personal meanings.

There was a man in the square today
He had a megaphone
But I didn't want to hear him
Yet he invaded my ears and
Penetrated my brain in a most peculiar way
I wanted to yell at him
To tell him to shut up
Get out of my ears,my head, my mind
But do you think he listened?
No
Give me peace, give me freedom
Give me sacred silence!
And still he kept on shouting
Edging the sanity out of my mind
Why can't he whisper or just holler at someone else?
Bursting my eardrums with noise so intense
Can't make out what he's saying
What's the point of all of this?
Madness softly creeps up on me
Ready to ambush me
To steal my rationality
To smash this unreality
And no-one can come and rescue me
Got to do it by myself
Ignore him and his megaphone
Is he really real anyway?
I just don't know.
But I say GO!

WHAT I SAW...........

This is all about seeing amazing visuals.

The sky is different today
Instead of being blue
A wonderful coloured array
A most unusual view
For it appears a chequerboard
has taken o'er the sky!
This simply cannot be ignored
A marvel way up high!

And on this chequerboard I see
Grey spheres made out of stone
And hewn so they sit perfectly
On their chequerboard home
I see beyond the rainbow's end
To the edge of the universe
And contemplate this world my friend
So happy I could burst!

I love this chequerboard sky so
I don't want to close my eyes
In case it should just up and go
Or clouds so dark disguise
Come! Look out of my window
And wonder at the sight!
But you shake your head, say no
That I can't be feeling right?

You say to me all serious
Did you take your medication?
And I become so furious
I don't want interrogation!
Your chequerboard sky- it isn't real
It's all just an illusion
Please don't tell me how to feel
Don't say it's a delusion!
For how I loved that wondrous sight
That stretched across the sky

Tales from a Broken Mind

I hope it comes again one night
I wish, I hope, I sigh
But if it has been lost forever
Then forever shall I mourn
The sight some thought was never ever
The sight I saw at dawn.

QUESTIONS

Another one about Mr Sarky.

As I contemplate this
Tear drops sting my eyes
Always seeking answers
But only hearing lies.

I have burning questions
Issues puzzling me
I need to hear the truth
For that will set me free.

No more lame excuses
It's not me it's you
I am not that stupid
Now tell me something true!

DON'T GIVE UP...........

This is one all about how I try to help other people going through
similar experiences to me and how I try to keep hope alive for these
people.

You sit there swathed in sadness
The bluest of the blue
You've been embraced by madness
And that my friend is true.

Tears course down your cheeks now
It makes you wish for death
But you'll get through this somehow
As long as you have breath

Although life seems so stark
You feel your future's bleak
A glimmer that lights up the dark
Your voice finds words to speak

For though you think that I'm strong
Well, I was once like you
The journey and the fight were long
But see- I made it through.

So wipe away those tears friend
Never admit defeat
Now's the beginning-not the end
Remember, life is sweet!

SELF INFLICTED PAIN

This is a kind of cautionary tale about how no matter what voices
tell you, self-harm is never the answer.

For all the things they did to you
There's one thing you must see
And that is self-inflicted pain
Will never set you free

For all those ghastly memories
The things they said to you
Remember self inflicted pain
Won't help you see what's true

For all the things they should have done
Your needs they did neglect
Stop! As self-inflicted pain
Won't gain you their respect

For all those lonely nights you cried
From frustration and hurt
Please see that self-inflicted pain
Won't improve your self-worth

For you are worth much more than that
So keep that thought in mind
You don't need self-inflicted pain
To leave the past behind

Keep walking forth into the light
And reaching for the stars
Goodbye to self-inflicted pain
No need to add more scars.

SCAR STORY

This is all about the scars I have on my body from self-harming because of the things Mr Sarky has said to me and how each one tells a story of how I survived despite all the problems I have experienced.

This one's for the creep that tried
To pull a move on me
And this one's for an argument
The point I failed to see.
This one's for the nasty words
The years of hard neglect
And this one's for the silent tears
The bitterest regret.
This one's for the loneliness
The years of isolation
And this one's for the ignorance
A lifetime of frustration.
This one's for the things he said
And tried to make me do
This one's for the lies he told
Nothing he said was true.
This one's for the weakness
When I should have been strong
The nights I felt too scared to sleep
In case it all went wrong.
But this one's most significant
Of all upon my arm
It marks the very last time
That my own skin I did harm

PANIC ATTACK

This is pretty self-explanatory. It is all about how it feels to have a
panic attack.

Walking down the street
Everything's normal
Everything's fine.
Minding my own business
And it's all right
It's all okay.
A spring in my step
Very good, yes
It's very nice.
And then it happens.
They're watching me.
Laughing at me.
I can even hear them saying things
Nasty things.
Evil things.
I feel the panic rising
Consuming me
Devouring me.
Heart pounding, head thumping
Get a grip!
Sort it out!
But THEY want to kill me
See me dead.
See me gone.
I can hear their twisted thoughts
They hate me.
Despise me.
My face is red, my palms sweaty.
Give me air!
Need some air!
So I turn back and run home
Another failure.
Another mistake.
Indoors now and the tears come
I'm useless.
Feel hopeless.

Tales from a Broken Mind

Maybe I'll just stay in
Can't go outside
I can't face it.
But the voices are still there.
Laughing at me.
Taunting me.
And there is no escape
From my own head
From myself.
But life goes on out there
Either with me
Or without me.
And as I drift off to sleep now
The pain-it fades
I am free.............

ANGEL OR.....DEMON?

A bit of an angry one! Aimed at Mr Sarky and his constant barrage of lies.

Look into my eyes
And tell me what you see
An angel or a demon
Which is most like me?

I hope that you say
That you can't see either
As I am only human
Good or bad or neither!

You wouldn't see the truth
So please don't be surprised
That I still feel angry
When you had me exorcised!

For I was just unwell
I wasn't turning bad
I really needed help then
Felt like I was going mad.

I wish you could have seen it
How I was feeling broken
And helped me when I needed it
Possessed? You must be joking!

BLAH, BLAH, BLAH.

This all about the stuff Mr Sarky tells me and how when I am
feeling relatively well, I can dismiss it for what it is-rubbish!

Blah, blah, blah
I've heard it all before
So please don't try to bore me
By saying it some more!

Blah, blah, blah
You think that you know best
But I don't heed what you say
So just give it a rest!

Blah, blah, blah
You're always telling me
That you know it much better
Someone! Set me free!

Blah, blah, blah
You're going on and on
Stick my fingers in my ears
Hey presto! You have gone!

Blah, blah, blah
Just watch me walk away
Can't be bothered with you now
I don't care what you say!

NOT SO SMART

Another one about Mr Sarky.

You think that you know best
Now let's just wait and see
You may live to regret
Arguing with me!
You might have the answers
But I think I must say
Not as smart as you think
Now please just go away!
No-one likes a know-all
Really most annoying
I'll wait for you to hush
And peace- I'll be enjoying!

REMEMBER

A self-explanatory poem about being written off as a child by adults
who should have known better.

Remember how you wrote me off
Think back, do you recall?
Even though I was so young
Just a child at school.

How you said I would not go far
My hopes and dreams you dashed
I'm glad I didn't listen
Your cruel words I smashed.

Well, I've got news for you my dear
Things are good and it's true
I pay no heed to judgements
From bigots such as you!

MISS YOU............

This is all about my Grandmother and how she supported me so much through my worst days. I feel bad as she is now in a nursing home and suffering from dementia. It is a cruel disease and I wish I could help her in the way she helped me.

Oh I never knew that I
Relied on you so much
It's only now I realise
Now we're not in touch.

You helped me so much back then
To heal my broken mind
But now I'm sad to say it
Those days so far behind.

I wish that I could help you
The way that you helped me
But nothing that I can do
Will ever set you free.

Your body weak and ravaged
And your mind is shattered
Now I cling to memories
For they are all that matter.

I won't forget your wise words
Nor lose sight of your smile
Because you knew just what to say
When I found life quite vile.

But now you sit and fade away
Just turn and face the light,
For all that you have done for me
I won't give up my fight.

HOPE FADES......

This is all about feeling that there is no hope and then seeing that there is!

Now the fading sun flickers
As do my dreams
The laughter I once had
Has now turned to screams

No hope on the horizon
I strain my eyes
The joy that I always had
Is replaced by my cries.

I wish I could reach out now
But no-one's there
Stuck in sad silence
With damage to repair.

Will the light return again?
I really don't know
Ravaged by my doubt
I can't see where to go.

This fog has descended
And there is no light
Stealing away sound
And obscuring my sight.

But you will never beat me
Nor push me to the ground
For though I was once lost
Now I have been found!

NINE O'CLOCK...........

This is all about a coping strategy I use. It's called the 'Nine O'
Clock Rule'. Basically I tell Mr Sarky that I am too busy to talk to
him at the moment he chooses to speak to me. I then tell him that I
will speak to him at nine o' clock and that he will have ten minutes
in which to say what he wants to say and I can tell him what I think
of him. It is very effective as he rarely bothers to show up!!!

Ok so you're there.
I can hear you
I'm aware!
But must you plague me so?
You never seem to let up
You're always in my ear!
So just go away!
I need a break
And today!
But no- you have to push me
To the edge of my temper
And beyond sometimes
Now leave me alone
I don't need you
So go home!
Your 'wit and your wisdom'
Don't cut it with me
As I know you're lying!
Just give me time
All on my own
It's a crime!
Why don't you get the message?
You're not welcome
I didn't invite you
Into my life
But there you are
Like a knife
Stuck in my side.
And you're twisted-you're warped!
I'd like to strangle you
So please hear me...
Get out my face

Tales from a Broken Mind

I don't like you
In my space
You can speak to me
When I ask you to
And absolutely not before!
So just take it
And go now
You faked it
Too many times and
I see right through you.
So get gone now unwelcome one!
Go away please
Hear me say
Not on my knees
Well, not today.
But you persist to exist
Crawl back under your stone
Leave well alone
I don't want you
Nor your dulcet tone!
Go away- Give me time
If I choose to
We'll speak at nine........

SNIPPETS...

This is a poem composed entirely of snippets of other people's conversations.

Oh good grief-don't say you did?
Please tell me that you never...
Angie's having Jonny's kid?
My dog is so damned clever!

No way! No-that can't be true!
Ronan's seeing Isabelle?
No- I am not speaking to you
Poor Jean-she's so unwell.

But I'm the one who's with Mark!
Never speak to a stranger!
Mummy I don't like the dark.
Behind the wheel she's a danger!

Know the film-Easy Rider?
Courtney- get here now!
In the bath -a huge spider!
I hate Jess-she's such a cow!

Gemma's with Jenny's hubby?
That's enough- no fighting!
Can I help with that luvvie?
Wow what awful hand-writing!

Can you all just sit still please!
What are you crying for?
Jamie-get up off your knees!
Mind your fingers with that door!

Come on now-it's time to go!
Let's all head for home.
I hope that you enjoyed the show!
Please don't feel alone!

FEELINGS.......

I wrote this one when I was feeling very low and depressed. It reflects the despair that depression can make you feel.

I feel the shame
It hurts my fragile heart
Tired of this game
Tearing me apart

I feel the guilt
It makes me feel so sad
I begin to wilt
Ev'rything seems bad

I feel the pain
It rips through my being
Driving me insane
Stopping me seeing

I feel the hate
It savages my soul
I am in a state
Losing my control

I feel despair
It really gets me down
Wish I didn't care
Silence all around

DOCTOR........

I wrote this one when I was feeling very angry about doctors not really listening to me and thinking that medication is the answer to everything.

Doctor, I'm having trouble sleeping
Feel so low I can't stop weeping.

Ok, could I have a description
Before I write you a prescription?

But I don't want your pills and powders!
Good grief! The voices are getting louder!

Now come on, won't you take your meds?
They're there to help you sort your head!

I see no harm in how I'm thinking
Really Doc- have you been drinking?

But can't you see that you are ill?
Do as you're told now- take that pill!

I'm sorry Doc, but no can do,
They might just cause my brain to stew!

Lightning Source UK Ltd.
Milton Keynes UK
UKOW04f1918170815

257087UK00001B/19/P